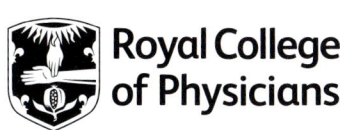 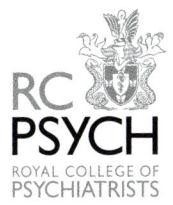 

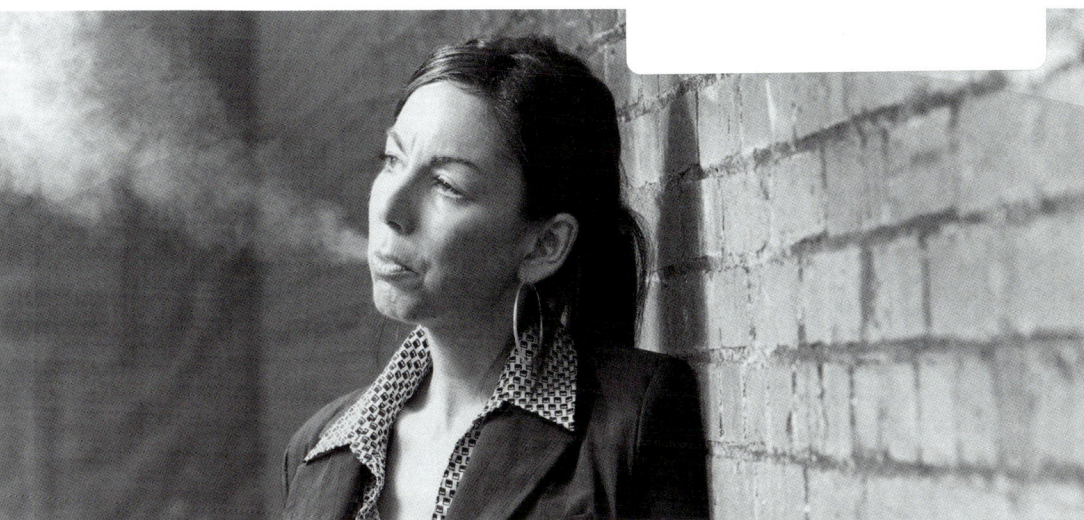

Smoking and mental health

A joint report by the Royal College of Physicians and the Royal College of Psychiatrists

Endorsed by:

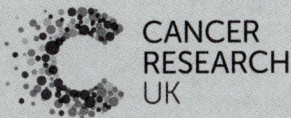 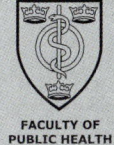

Acknowledgments

The Tobacco Advisory Group acknowledges with thanks contributions to the production of this report by staff and students at the UK Centre for Tobacco Control Studies (**www.ukctcs.org**), which is supported by core funding from the British Heart Foundation, Cancer Research UK, the Economic and Social Research Council, Medical Research Council and Department of Health under the auspices of the UK Clinical Research Collaboration. We thank Cancer Research UK for additional funding to support the systematic reviews and new data analyses, and EPIC for providing THIN data. We also thank Kapka Nilan for help in preparing bibliographies, and Joanna Reid and Urooj Asif Akhtar of the RCP Corporate Communications and Publishing team, for the production of this report.

The Royal College of Physicians

The Royal College of Physicians plays a leading role in the delivery of high-quality patient care by setting standards of medical practice and promoting clinical excellence. We provide physicians in over 30 medical specialties with education, training and support throughout their careers. As an independent charity representing more than 28,000 fellows and members worldwide, we advise and work with government, patients, allied healthcare professionals and the public to improve health and healthcare.

The Royal College of Psychiatrists

The Royal College of Psychiatrists is an independent charity that represents over 16,000 members worldwide. It exists to set standards and promote excellence in psychiatry and mental healthcare; to lead, represent and support psychiatrists; and to work with mental healthcare service users, carers and their organisations in achieving these aims.

Citation for this document

Royal College of Physicians, Royal College of Psychiatrists. *Smoking and mental health*. London: RCP, 2013.
Royal College of Psychiatrists Council Report CR178.

Copyright

All rights reserved. No part of this publication may be reproduced in any form (including photocopying or storing it in any medium by electronic means and whether or not transiently or incidentally to some other use of this publication) without the written permission of the copyright owner. Applications for the copyright owner's written permission to reproduce any part of this publication should be addressed to the publisher.

Copyright © Royal College of Physicians 2013

ISBN 978 1 86016 508 5
eISBN 978 1 86016 509 2

Royal College of Physicians
11 St Andrews Place
Regent's Park
London NW1 4LE
www.rcplondon.ac.uk
Registered Charity No 210508

Royal College of Psychiatrists
17 Belgrave Square
London SW1X 8PG
www.rcpsych.ac.uk
Registered Charity No 228636

Typeset by Cambrian Typesetters, Camberley, Surrey
Printed by The Lavenham Press Limited, Suffolk

Contents

Members of the Tobacco Advisory Group		x
Contributors		xi
Foreword		xiv

1 Mental disorders — 1
- 1.1 What is a mental disorder? — 1
- 1.2 Occurrence and associations of mental disorder — 2
- 1.3 Common mental disorders — 3
- 1.4 Other non-psychotic disorders — 3
  - 1.4.1 Obsessive–compulsive disorder — 3
  - 1.4.2 Post-traumatic stress disorder — 4
  - 1.4.3 Eating disorders — 4
  - 1.4.4 Somatisation disorder — 5
- 1.5 Psychotic disorders — 6
  - 1.5.1 Schizophrenia — 6
  - 1.5.2 Bipolar disorder — 7
- 1.6 Personality disorder — 7
- 1.7 Childhood disorders — 8
  - 1.7.1 Attention deficit hyperactivity disorder — 8
  - 1.7.2 Conduct disorders — 9
- 1.8 Dementia — 10
- 1.9 Mental health services — 11
- 1.10 Summary — 12

2 Smoking among people with mental disorders — 16
- 2.1 Introduction — 16
- 2.2 Data and methods — 16
  - 2.2.1 Health Survey for England — 16
  - 2.2.2 Adult Psychiatric Morbidity Survey — 17
  - 2.2.3 The Health Improvement Network — 19
- 2.3 Smoking prevalence — 21
  - 2.3.1 HSE — 21
  - 2.3.2 APMS — 22
  - 2.3.3 THIN — 23

2.4	Population estimates	25
2.5	Variations in smoking prevalence among those with mental disorder by age, sex and socioeconomic status	27
2.6	Strength of addiction	27
2.7	Association between cigarette consumption and mental disorders	29
2.8	Proportion of cigarettes smoked by people with a mental disorder	29
2.9	Quitting behaviour	29
2.10	Delivery of smoking cessation interventions	33
2.11	Supplementary APMS survey data on special populations	35
2.12	Summary	35

3 Neurobiological and behavioural mechanisms linking smoking and mental disorders — **38**

- 3.1 Mechanisms of nicotine addiction — 38
- 3.2 Models of association and sources of evidence — 39
  - 3.2.1 Genetic evidence — 40
  - 3.2.2 Animal models — 40
  - 3.2.3 Social and psychosocial mechanisms — 41
- 3.3 Depression and anxiety — 41
  - 3.3.1 Evidence from genetic studies — 42
  - 3.3.2 Evidence from animal studies — 42
  - 3.3.3 Evidence from human studies — 44
- 3.4 Schizophrenia — 46
  - 3.4.1 Evidence from genetic studies — 46
  - 3.4.2 Evidence from animal studies — 47
  - 3.4.3 Evidence from human studies — 47
- 3.5 Attention deficit hyperactivity disorder — 48
  - 3.5.1 Evidence from genetic studies — 48
  - 3.5.2 Evidence from animal studies — 49
  - 3.5.3 Evidence from human studies — 50
- 3.6 Smoking and dementia — 51
- 3.7 Future studies — 52
- 3.8 Summary — 52

4 Epidemiology of the association between smoking and mental disorders — **63**

- 4.1 Introduction — 63
- 4.2 Search methods — 63
- 4.3 Smoking and onset of any mental disorder — 64
- 4.4 Smoking and developmental and emotional disorders — 65
  - 4.4.1 Composite measures of behavioural and emotional disorders — 65
  - 4.4.2 Internalising and externalising problems — 66

		4.4.3	Attention deficit hyperactivity disorder	66
		4.4.4	Oppositional defiant disorder	67
		4.4.5	Conduct disorder	67
	4.5	Smoking and bipolar disorder		68
	4.6	Smoking and schizophrenia		69
	4.7	Smoking and anxiety disorders		70
	4.8	Smoking and eating disorders		70
	4.9	Smoking and depression		71
		4.9.1	Smoking and onset of depression	71
		4.9.2	Depression and onset of smoking	72
	4.10	Smoking and dementia		75
	4.11	Smoking and increased mortality and morbidity among people with mental disorders		76
	4.12	Summary		76

Appendix to Chapter 4 (Tables A1–7) is available online at **www.rcplondon.ac.uk/publications/smoking-and-mental-health**

5 Smoking cessation interventions for individuals with mental disorders — **84**

	5.1	General considerations		84
	5.2	Cessation interventions for severe mental illness		85
		5.2.1	Behavioural support	85
		5.2.2	Nicotine replacement therapy	86
		5.2.3	Bupropion	87
		5.2.4	Varenicline	87
		5.2.5	Cautions on use of bupropion and varenicline	88
	5.3	Cutting down on smoking, and other harm reduction strategies		89
		5.3.1	Behavioural interventions	89
		5.3.2	Nicotine replacement therapy	90
		5.3.3	Bupropion	90
		5.3.4	Varenicline	90
	5.4	Is it safe for people with SMI to give up smoking?		90
		5.4.1	Adverse events relating to smoking cessation interventions	91
		5.4.2	Effects of smoking cessation on mental health symptoms	91
		5.4.3	Weight gain	92
		5.4.4	Interactions with treatment for mental disorders	92
		5.4.5	Interactions with caffeine	95
		5.4.6	Nicotine withdrawal symptoms	95
		5.4.7	Effects of antipsychotic medication on smoking cessation	95

5.5		Provision of smoking cessation and tobacco dependence treatment for smokers with mental disorders in the UK	96
	5.5.1	Primary care	96
	5.5.2	Specialist mental health settings (secondary care)	97
	5.5.3	Child and adolescent mental health services	98
	5.5.4	NHS stop smoking services	99
	5.5.5	Enhancing service provision for smokers with mental disorders	100
5.6		Experience of attempts to introduce comprehensive smoking cessation support in mental health settings: UK case studies	100
	5.6.1	London, UK	100
	5.6.2	Nottingham, UK	101
	5.6.3	Implications for practice	103
5.7		Summary	103

6 Population strategies to prevent smoking in mental disorders — 111

6.1		Introduction	111
6.2		General population strategies	111
	6.2.1	Smoke-free legislation	111
	6.2.2	Mass media campaigns	112
	6.2.3	Health warnings	112
	6.2.4	Ending tobacco advertising, promotion and sponsorship	113
	6.2.5	Price increases	113
	6.2.6	Illicit tobacco	114
	6.2.7	Minimum legal age for cigarette purchase	114
	6.2.8	Smoking cessation services	114
	6.2.9	Preventing smoking uptake through school-based interventions	115
	6.2.10	Harm reduction	115
6.3		Population strategies and smoking prevention in mental health	116
	6.3.1	Smoke-free policies in mental health treatment settings	116
	6.3.2	Media campaigns	119
	6.3.3	Health warnings, advertising and sponsorship	119
	6.3.4	Price and illicit supply	119
	6.3.5	Minimum legal age of purchase	120
	6.3.6	NHS stop smoking services	120
	6.3.7	Harm reduction strategies	120
	6.3.8	School-based interventions	120
6.4		Factors perpetuating smoking in mental health settings	121
	6.4.1	A smoking culture	121
	6.4.2	Staff beliefs and attitudes	121

		6.4.3	Staff knowledge	122
		6.4.4	Staff smoking	122
		6.4.5	Systems, targets, and resources	123
	6.5	Summary		124

7 Smoking and mental disorders: special circumstances — 130

	7.1	Forensic psychiatric inpatient services		130
		7.1.1	Introduction	130
		7.1.2	Smoking prevalence in forensic psychiatric services	131
		7.1.3	Smoking cessation support within forensic psychiatric services	131
		7.1.4	Smoke-free policies in forensic psychiatric services	131
		7.1.5	Maintaining a smoke-free environment	133
		7.1.6	Summary points	134
	7.2	Prisons		134
		7.2.1	Introduction	134
		7.2.2	Smoking and mental disorders in prison populations	135
		7.2.3	Smoke-free policy in prisons	136
		7.2.4	Effectiveness and uptake of cessation services in prisons	137
		7.2.5	Design of prison cessation services	137
		7.2.6	Regime issues	138
		7.2.7	Staff attitudes and logistics	138
		7.2.8	Misuse of NRT	139
		7.2.9	Impact of mental disorders in the prison setting	139
		7.2.10	Summary points	139
	7.3	Smoking and misuse of alcohol or other drugs		140
		7.3.1	Prevalence of alcohol and drug misuse	140
		7.3.2	Smoking and alcohol or drug misuse	140
		7.3.3	Mental disorders and alcohol or drug misuse	141
		7.3.4	Impact of smoking in people with alcohol or drug misuse	141
		7.3.5	Smoking cessation and alcohol or drug misuse	142
		7.3.6	Summary points	143
	7.4	Homeless people		143
		7.4.1	The size of the UK homeless population	143
		7.4.2	Homelessness and mental disorders	143
		7.4.3	Smoking and homelessness	144
		7.4.4	Excess mortality and health service use among homeless people	144
		7.4.5	Smoking cessation in homeless people	145
		7.4.6	Increasing smoking cessation in homeless people	145
		7.4.7	Summary points	146
	7.5	Smoking, mental disorders and pregnancy		146
		7.5.1	Smoking in pregnancy	146

	7.5.2	Mental disorders and smoking in pregnancy	147
	7.5.3	Smoking cessation in pregnancy	147
	7.5.4	Smoking cessation in pregnant women with mental disorders	147
	7.5.5	Summary points	148
7.6		Children and adolescents	149
	7.6.1	Prenatal smoking and mental health in children and young people	149
	7.6.2	Passive smoking and mental health in children and young people	149
	7.6.3	Smoking and child and adolescent mental disorders	150
	7.6.4	Looked-after children and smoking	151
	7.6.5	Smoking prevention and cessation in children and adolescents with mental disorders and in looked-after children	152
	7.6.6	Summary points	153
7.7		Special circumstances summary	153

8	**The economic cost of smoking in people with mental disorders**		**164**
8.1	Introduction		164
8.2	Estimating the costs of diseases caused by smoking in people with mental disorders		164
8.3	Hospital costs of treating disease caused by smoking in people with mental disorders		165
8.4	Outpatient services and primary care		169
8.5	Cost savings from psychotropic drug dose reduction after smoking cessation		171
8.6	Life-years gained from smoking cessation in mental disorders		173
8.7	Harm reduction approaches		176
8.8	Summary		178

9	**Ethical and legal aspects**	**182**
9.1	Context	182
9.2	Legal precedents	183
9.3	Population and individual arguments	184
9.4	Access to treatment for smoking	186
9.5	Summary	187

10	**Overall conclusions**	**189**
10.1	Smoking in Britain	189
10.2	Mental disorders and smoking in Britain	189
10.3	The nature of the association between smoking and mental disorders	190
10.4	Smoking cessation in mental disorders	191

	10.5	Tobacco policy and mental health	191
	10.6	Special circumstances	192
	10.7	Economic costs of smoking in people with mental disorders	193
	10.8	Ethics	193
	10.9	Research priorities	194
11	**Key conclusions and recommendations**		**195**

Members of the Tobacco Advisory Group of the Royal College of Physicians

Deborah Arnott

Richard Ashcroft

John Britton (Chair)

Jonathan Campion*

Tim Coleman

Linda Cuthbertson

Anna Gilmore

Louise Howard*

Allan Hackshaw

Martin Jarvis

Jo Leonardi-Bee

Andrew McCracken

Ann McNeill

Jennifer Percival

Elena Ratschen*

---

*Co-opted for the production of this report.

Contributors

Anthony Aclet – Specialist stop smoking advisor/physical health lead, South West London and St George's Mental Health NHS Trust

Richard Ashcroft – Professor of bioethics, Queen Mary University of London

David Balfour – Emeritus professor of behavioural pharmacology, University of Dundee

Lindsay Banham – Academic clinical fellow in psychiatry, Institute of Psychiatry, King's College London

Michelle Baybutt – Research & development coordinator, Healthy Settings Unit, University of Central Lancashire

John Britton – Professor of epidemiology, UK Centre for Tobacco Control Studies, University of Nottingham

Jonathan Campion – Director for public mental health and consultant psychiatrist, South London and Maudsley NHS Foundation Trust

Irene Cormac – Honorary consultant forensic psychiatrist, Rampton Hospital, Nottinghamshire Healthcare NHS Trust

Suzy Dymond-White – Tobacco policy lead, National Offender Management Service

Tamsin Ford – Clinical senior lecturer, University of Exeter Medical School

Simon Gilbody – Professor of psychological medicine and health services research, University of York

Allan Hackshaw – Professor of epidemiology and medical statistics, Cancer Research UK & UCL Cancer Trials Centre, Cancer Institute, University College London

Alex Higgins – Specialist stop smoking advisor, Sidmouth, Devon

Matthew Hotopf – Professor of general hospital psychiatry, Institute of Psychiatry, King's College London

Louise Howard – Professor of women's mental health, Institute of Psychiatry, King's College London

Martin Jarvis – Emeritus professor of health psychology, University College London

David Kalman – Associate professor of psychiatry, University of Massachusetts, USA

Jo Leonardi-Bee – Associate professor of medical statistics, UK Centre for Tobacco Control Studies, University of Nottingham

Susan MacAskill – Senior researcher, Institute for Social Marketing, University of Stirling and Open University, Stirling

Mei-See Man – Research fellow, School of Social and Community Medicine, University of Bristol

Lisa McNally – Public health principal, NHS Surrey

Ann McNeill – Professor of tobacco addiction, UK Centre for Tobacco Control Studies, King's College London

Marcus Munafò – Professor of biological psychology, UK Centre for Tobacco Control Studies, University of Bristol

Tamsin Newlove-Delgado – Specialty registrar in public health, NHS Devon; Honorary university fellow, University of Exeter Medical School

Camilla Parker – Research assistant, UK Centre for Tobacco Control Studies, University of Nottingham

Steve Parrott – Senior research fellow, UK Centre for Tobacco Control Studies, Department of Health Sciences, University of York

Hembadoon Piné-Abata – Postgraduate student, University of Nottingham

Elena Ratschen – Lecturer in epidemiology/tobacco control, UK Centre for Tobacco Control Studies, University of Nottingham

Melissa Rowe – Academic clinical fellow in obstetrics and gynaecology, University College London

Lisa Szatkowski – Lecturer in medical statistics, UK Centre for Tobacco Control Studies, University of Nottingham

Gillian Shorter – Lecturer in mental health sciences, University of Ulster

Robert Stewart – Professor of psychiatric epidemiology and clinical informatics, Institute of Psychiatry, King's College London

Catherine Whittington – Medical student, University of Nottingham

Jill Williams – Associate professor in psychiatry, UMDNJ-Robert Wood Johnson Medical School, New Jersey, USA

Qi Wu – Research fellow, Department of Health Sciences, University of York

Douglas M. Ziedonis – Professor and chair, Department of Psychiatry, University of Massachusetts Medical School and UMass Memorial Health Care, USA

Foreword

Smoking is the largest direct avoidable cause of death and disability, and the largest cause of inequalities in health, in the UK. Since 1962, when the Royal College of Physicians (RCP) published its first report on smoking and health, the prevalence of smoking in the UK has fallen dramatically, but not in all sectors of society. As a result, smoking is becoming the domain of the most disadvantaged: the poor, the unemployed, the homeless, the imprisoned and the mentally ill. Of the 10 million smokers in the UK today, almost one in three reports mental health problems. The prevalence of smoking among people with mental disorders has barely changed in the past 20 years. This is an indictment of UK public health policy and clinical service provision.

This report describes and quantifies the burden of disease caused by smoking in people with mental disorders, and identifies ways in which health professionals, and particularly doctors, can provide the leadership necessary to change the prevailing culture of acceptance and perpetuation of smoking in this group. As smoking becomes less prevalent in our society, so the need to identify and reverse failures of health policy and service provision for those who remain dependent on tobacco smoking becomes more urgent. This report calls for radical changes in the prioritisation, service provision and prevention of this major cause of premature death and disability in people with mental disorders.

It is an area in which change is long overdue.

Sir Richard Thompson
President, Royal College of Physicians

Sue Bailey
President, Royal College of Psychiatrists

Lindsey Davies
President, Faculty of Public Health

1 Mental disorders

1.1 What is a mental disorder?

Mental health problems, referred to in this report as mental disorders, are common in the general population and include depressive and anxiety disorders, eating and somatisation disorders, and psychotic disorders (schizophrenia, bipolar disorder and related disorders such as schizoaffective psychosis). Different mental disorders are characterised by different symptoms (see sections 1.3–1.8) and are defined less by the occurrence of specific symptoms (subjective complaints) or signs (behaviours) than by their severity or clustering to the extent that causes distress and interference with personal function.[1] The distinction of depression from ordinary sadness, or schizophrenia from the paranoid delusional thinking and auditory hallucinations that occur in up to 8% of healthy people,[2] is somewhat arbitrary, as indeed is the case in other areas of medicine, eg in determining the levels of blood pressure or blood sugar that define hypertension or diabetes. Indeed, some mental health research and clinical practice involve use of self-report symptom scales with different cut-offs used to distinguish probable mild disorders from more severe disorders. However, the use of binary distinctions to differentiate disorder from normality is common to most areas of medicine and reflects the importance of clinical diagnoses in guiding healthcare planning, and the delivery of prognostic and treatment advice in clinical management.

For mental disorders, the main internationally recognised diagnostic classifications currently in use are the World Heath Organization's (WHO's) *International classification of diseases*, 10th revision (ICD-10)[1] and the American *Diagnostic and statistical manual of mental disorders*, 4th edition (DSM-IV),[3] both of which are currently being revised and updated (to ICD-11 and DSM-V respectively). The term 'mental disorder' in these classifications also includes personality disorder (see below), dementia (a degenerative disorder that is usually treated within mental health services and is included in this report), and alcohol and drug disorders and nicotine dependence. Primary alcohol and substance misuse disorders are not specifically addressed in this report because they are beyond its scope, but they are also associated with smoking and are discussed in the context of co-morbidity with other primary mental disorders. However, co-morbid alcohol and substance misuse, as well as smoking, is extremely common in those with other mental disorders.

1.2 Occurrence and associations of mental disorder

About a quarter of the population experience some form of mental disorder, most commonly mild and self-limiting depression or anxiety, in any one year.[4] Psychotic disorders are much less common – a recent review of studies in England reported that around 0.4% of the population had an active psychotic disorder in the past year.[5] Psychotic disorders are sometimes referred to as 'serious mental illnesses', although severe forms of non-psychotic disorders such as depression or obsessive–compulsive disorder can be similarly disabling.

All mental disorders, but particularly mood disorders and schizophrenia, are associated with an increased risk of suicide.[6] Mental disorders are socially stigmatised and, as a result, people with mental disorders, particularly those with severe conditions, can experience discrimination and a sense of being shunned by society.[7] This stigma can lead to impoverishment, social marginalisation and low quality of life,[8] and to discrimination in access to and quality of services for physical illness.[9] People with mental disorders are also more likely to live in circumstances of socioeconomic deprivation, partly as a result of deprivation playing a role in the causal pathway to disorder (the stress-vulnerability model), and partly because the disorder itself can lead to loss of employment, housing, income and other attributes. The relative importance of these directional models differs for different disorders, with deprivation appearing to be a strong cause of depression, for example,[10] whereas the association with schizophrenia is largely due to the illness leading to worsening of socioeconomic circumstances.[11] This relationship with deprivation is also likely to impact on the prevalence of smoking in people with mental disorders, because smoking is strongly associated with socioeconomic deprivation.

There is increasing recognition that people with mental disorders are at increased risk of adverse physical health outcomes, to the extent that people with severe mental illness have a substantially lower life expectancy. A recent study in south London found that having a psychiatric diagnosis was associated with a loss of at least 8 life-years for men, and 10 for women, with particularly high reductions for men with schizophrenia (14.6 years lost) and women with schizoaffective disorders (17.5 years lost).[12] This loss of life appears to be largely due to cardiovascular disease,[13] for which smoking is one of the main risk factors.[14] Smoking is a common, under-treated and under-recognised problem in this patient population.[15]

1.3 Common mental disorders

Depression and anxiety are common mental disorders, with a lifetime prevalence of at least 25%.[4] Depression, defined as a disorder if symptoms have been present for at least 2 weeks, is the most common; symptoms include feeling sad or irritable most of the time, loss of pleasure or interest in things that used to be enjoyed, significant loss or gain of weight that is unrelated to physical illness or pregnancy, difficulty sleeping or over-sleeping, feeling restless or slowed down, fatigue, feelings of worthlessness or excessive guilt, and difficulties concentrating, remembering or making decisions. There may be thoughts of self-harm or suicide. Depressive disorders can also be associated with prominent symptoms of anxiety. Risk factors for depression include younger age, female gender, low educational achievement, a previous history of depression, a family history of depression, childhood maltreatment and adulthood domestic violence.[16–18] Less commonly, severe depression occurs with psychotic symptoms and is then classified as an affective (mood-related) psychotic disorder (see below).

Anxiety disorders include phobias such as agoraphobia (fear and avoidance of crowds, public places or travelling away from home), social phobia (marked fear of being the focus of attention, fear of behaving in a way that will be embarrassing, and marked avoidance of situations in which there is fear of behaving in an embarrassing way), panic disorder (recurrent panic attacks) and generalised anxiety disorder (at least 6 months of prominent tension, worry and feelings of apprehension about everyday events and problems, with anxiety symptoms). Anxiety symptoms include autonomic arousal symptoms (eg palpitations, sweating, trembling, dry mouth), difficulty in breathing, and fear of dying or losing control.[1]

The 2007 Adult Psychiatric Morbidity Survey (APMS) in England found that women were more likely than men to have a common mental disorder (19.7% and 12.5% respectively), and that this applied for all disorder categories except panic and obsessive–compulsive disorder.[4] Depression and anxiety tend to be recurrent or persistent in most patients.[19]

1.4 Other non-psychotic disorders

1.4.1 Obsessive–compulsive disorder

Obsessive–compulsive disorder (OCD) is characterised by the presence of obsessions (unwanted intrusive thoughts, images or urges, which repeatedly enter the person's mind) or compulsions (repetitive behaviours or mental acts that the person feels driven to perform, such as checking that taps are switched off, or repeatedly cleaning), and commonly both. OCD occurs in around 1% of people,[20] with similar rates in men and women, and may follow an acute, episodic or chronic course. In one 40-year follow-up study, only 20% of patients experienced full remission, although approximately 60% displayed signs of general improvement;[21] however, other studies have found better outcomes.[22] Risk factors include adverse life events and a family history of OCD.[23]

1.4.2 Post-traumatic stress disorder

Post-traumatic stress disorder (PTSD) develops after exposure to trauma and includes re-experiencing symptoms, flashbacks in which the person acts or feels as if the event is recurring, nightmares, hypervigilance, irritability, difficulty concentrating, sleep problems and avoidance of trauma. In the APMS, 3% of the adult population fulfilled criteria for PTSD with no significant difference by gender.[4] Risk factors include a previous personal or family history of anxiety disorders or affective disorders, neuroticism, low intelligence, female gender and a history of previous trauma.[18,24,25]

1.4.3 Eating disorders

Recent classifications have included three types of eating disorders: anorexia nervosa, which is characterised by extremely low bodyweight and a fear of weight gain, with restriction of food; bulimia nervosa, which is characterised by repeated binge eating, followed by behaviours to counteract it; and other eating disorders including binge eating without counteractive measures, and hence associated obesity.[1] In adults, the lifetime prevalence of eating disorders is around 0·6% for anorexia nervosa, 1% for bulimia nervosa and 3% for binge eating disorder. Women are three times more likely to be affected by these disorders than men, and prevalence decreases with age.

Anorexia nervosa typically lasts for about 6 years, with about 50% of patients experiencing a full recovery.[26] Factors associated with worse outcomes (including death) include the presence of other psychological symptoms and disorders, poor social functioning, longer duration of disease and substance abuse.[27] For bulimia nervosa, for which there is less information available on natural history, the outlook appears better, with resolution of symptoms in most patients and no evident increase in mortality.[28] Factors clearly associated with worse outcomes include depression, substance use and poor impulse control.[27] Common risk factors for eating disorders are female gender, white ethnicity (with some variation internationally), early childhood eating and gastrointestinal problems, elevated weight and shape concerns, negative self-evaluation, sexual abuse and other adverse experiences, and general psychiatric morbidity.[29] However, the most potent risk factors appear to be critical comments about eating from a teacher, coach or siblings, and a history of depression.[30]

1.4.4 Somatisation disorder

Somatisation disorder is the most severe form of a group of conditions collectively known as somatoform disorders, in which the patient presents with a physical health complaint, the doctor fails to find a conventional physical cause and the reason for the presentation is thought to have a psychological basis. These are difficult conditions to diagnose and research because diagnosis is to a large extent a function of the interaction between doctor and patient. Defining when a complaint has a satisfactory biomedical explanation can be very difficult, and the diagnoses defined under the rubric of somatoform disorders are a somewhat arbitrary collection of presentations defined by the presence of symptoms (eg somatisation disorder), the presence of overwhelming and troubling beliefs that one is ill (eg hypochondriasis) or the loss of neurological function (eg conversion disorder). These disorders represent extreme manifestations of a major clinical problem faced by most medical disciplines: that of medically unexplained symptoms.

Medically unexplained symptoms are a universal experience[31] and are sometimes referred to as 'functional', indicating that they are caused by (reversible) alterations in the body's function rather than pathological changes. People with such symptoms may understandably become concerned and seek explanations and help in doing so.[32] Although such presentations may be an indication of an underlying psychiatric disorder, particularly anxiety or depression, not all are.[33] However, psychological processes are always important in understanding symptoms, and include perceptual processes related to the selective attention that a symptom is given, cognitive processes that might relate to the meaning that the patient puts on the symptoms, affective responses such as fear and behavioural processes such as avoidance. Hence someone might experience a headache, find it hard to ignore this, become anxious about it and perhaps attach a meaning that is understandable although incorrect (eg thinking 'maybe it's a brain tumour'), and respond by seeking help and taking time off work. Such individuals are readily treated using approaches such as cognitive–behavioural therapy.[34]

For individuals with somatisation disorder such symptoms come to dominate life. To diagnose the disorder, unexplained symptoms have to be present in several bodily symptoms, start before the age of 30 and cause significant disruption to life. DSM-IV requires the presence of four pain symptoms, two gastrointestinal symptoms, one sexual symptom and one pseudo-neurological symptom to make the diagnosis; however, these thresholds are somewhat arbitrary and there is a strong case for a so-called 'abridged' somatisation disorder which has fewer symptoms.[35] The condition is present in approximately 1% of the population, with a strong female preponderance and associations with abusive experiences in childhood, physical illness in a relative during childhood, and co-morbid depression or anxiety.[36] Patients typically go through life seeking help from multiple doctors, undergoing unnecessary interventions (eg surgery) and having severe occupational impairments. For the most severe patients the natural history is chronic and unremitting.[37]

1.5 Psychotic disorders

1.5.1 Schizophrenia

Schizophrenia is characterised by fundamental and characteristic distortions of thinking and perception, and an inappropriate or lack of emotional responsiveness. Clear consciousness and intellectual capacity are usually maintained, although cognitive deficits (difficulties in memory, attention and executive functioning) can develop over time. Delusions and hallucinatory voices discussing the patient, disorganised speech and negative symptoms (including marked apathy, paucity of speech and blunting or incongruity of emotional responses, which usually result in social withdrawal and lowering of social performance) can occur. Mood can also be affected with depressive or manic symptoms, although patients who have few negative symptoms and a high level of mood (depression or mania) symptoms are usually diagnosed with psychotic depression or bipolar disorder. Where symptoms of schizophrenia and mood disorder occur in the same episode, the diagnosis of schizoaffective disorder will usually be made, also depending on other features of the course of illness. Prognosis is better for schizoaffective disorder than for schizophrenia, but worse than mood disorders.

The incidence of schizophrenia is around 15/100,000 persons per year, more in men than women (incidence ratio 1.4:1).[38] Onset can be insidious with subtle alterations in behaviour (sometimes known as the prodrome), or may be abrupt with varying presentations including delusions and/or hallucinations, sleep disturbance and rapid deterioration in social functioning. There is considerable heterogeneity in outcome with around 15% of patients experiencing a single episode of illness, 20–30% experiencing an episodic course, and others experiencing severe chronic social or intellectual deficit and/or chronic continuous psychotic symptoms.[2] Men tend to have a poorer outcome and this is associated with an earlier age at onset, typically in adolescence or the early 20s. Although medication (antipsychotic drugs) is available for schizophrenia it is mainly effective in targeting 'positive' symptoms such as the hallucinations and delusions, rather than the more disabling (in the long term) 'negative symptoms' such as apathy and social withdrawal. Treatment of schizophrenia does not appear to have a major impact on long-term outcome.

There is strong evidence of a genetic component in the aetiology of schizophrenia; other risk factors include growing up in an urban environment, childhood adversity, immigrant ethnicity (particularly if for those living in a low ethnic density area, or an area where there are fewer people of the same migrant group) and cannabis use. There is increasing evidence for genetic moderation of environmental influences on disease occurrence.[2]

In addition to schizophrenia, other psychotic disorders include bipolar disorder (see below), psychotic depression, schizoaffective disorder and delusional disorders. Recent evidence suggests that between 2 and 3% of the population will experience a psychotic disorder at some point in their lifetime.[2]

1.5.2 Bipolar disorder

Bipolar disorder (formerly known as manic–depressive illness) is characterised by two or more episodes of intense emotional states in which mood and activity are substantially disturbed. On some occasions mood is elevated, and energy and activity increased (known as hypomania), or, when psychotic features are present, the illness is described as a manic episode. On other occasions mood is lowered, and energy and activity decreased (depression). Repeated episodes of mania or hypomania are classified as bipolar disorder I and II respectively. Lifetime prevalence estimates are 1.0% for bipolar disorder I and 1.1% for bipolar disorder II.[39] Bipolar disorder is equally prevalent among men and women, with the exception of rapid cycling, which is a severe and difficult-to-treat variant of the disorder in which four or more episodes occur during 12 months, and arises mostly in women.[40]

Bipolar disorder is a chronic disorder characterised by relapses. Up to 20% of individuals with bipolar disorder take their own life, and nearly a third of patients admit to at least one suicide attempt.[40] However, mood stabilisers can be very effective in preventing relapse. Risk factors include genetic vulnerability,[41] black and minority ethnicity,[42] and psychosocial stressors such as childhood abuse or neglect, which can also predict poor outcome.[43]

1.6 Personality disorder

The concept of personality disorder refers to personalities associated with functional impairment. The term therefore refers to characteristic, enduring and pervasive patterns of inner experience and behaviour that deviate markedly as a whole from the culturally expected and accepted range (or 'norm'). However, as with other areas of psychiatric classification, the categorical nature of diagnosis simplifies the dimensional nature of the underlying personality features. There are several different types of personality disorder, which are classified in the ICD-10 as paranoid, schizoid, dissocial, emotionally unstable (with subtypes of impulsive and borderline), histrionic, anxious, dependent and anankastic.[1] Many people have features of more than one type.

Personality disorders are common, with a community prevalence in the UK of 4.4%.[44] By definition, they significantly impair personal and social functioning, with considerable cost to the health service, the criminal justice system and the individual.[45] Personality disorders are associated with medical service use and medical morbidity and mortality, especially from cardiovascular disease.[46] Of the subtypes of personality disorder, borderline and antisocial (dissocial) disorders are the most prominent in forensic and general psychiatric settings.[45] Borderline personality disorder is characterised by volatile relationships, an unstable self-image, labile mood and impulsiveness with frequent self-harm. Antisocial personality disorder is characterised by breaking rules routinely, engaging in criminal behaviour, and a strong tendency to be reckless, irresponsible and deceitful. People with both disorders often report a history of serious family problems, domestic violence, abuse, and inconsistent and often violent punishment in childhood. Personality disorders are often associated with other psychiatric[45] disorders such as depression or substance misuse. Borderline personality disorder can also occur with other psychotic disorders, eating disorders and PTSD.[45] In the past, personality disorders were often thought to be untreatable, but although personality features are long lasting they are not necessarily permanent. Recent research suggests that psychological interventions can be helpful; different types of interventions have been studied for different personality disorders, with most research focusing on borderline personality disorder and antisocial personality disorder. The most robust evidence to date suggests that psychological interventions such as dialectical behaviour therapy and mentalisation-based therapy for borderline personality disorder are effective in improving mood and reducing self-harm.[47] The National Institute for Health and Clinical Excellence (NICE) also emphasises the treatment of co-morbid disorders, and the importance of establishing an optimistic and trusting relationship.[45]

1.7 Childhood disorders

Mental disorders in children and young people are sometimes categorised in two groups: internalising and externalising. Emotional disorders such as depression and anxiety are often referred to as 'internalising disorders', whereas disorders involving more disruptive behaviours such as attention deficit hyperactivity disorder (ADHD) and conduct disorder fall into the category of 'externalising disorders'.

1.7.1 Attention deficit hyperactivity disorder

Attention deficit hyperactivity disorder is a complex developmental disorder of childhood with UK prevalence estimates in school-aged children at around 2–3%,[48] although some estimates from the international literature are higher.[49] The core behaviours are inattention, hyperactivity and impulsiveness, which are developmentally inappropriate and cause significant impairment in functioning. Symptoms are usually evident before the age of 7, although sometimes they are not diagnosed until adulthood. ADHD symptoms decline with age, but can persist into adult life in up to 60% of cases.[50] It is estimated that worldwide around 2% of adults may be affected.[51] People with this disorder have a high level of psychiatric co-morbidity, and are more likely to underachieve educationally and occupationally, and to be unemployed.[52,53] Proposed risk factors include a genetic influence, very low birthweight,[54] maternal smoking, exposure to lead, and consumption of additives and preservatives in the diet.[55] A small proportion of children improve after alterations in their diet.[49]

1.7.2 Conduct disorders

Conduct disorders are characterised by repetitive patterns of antisocial, disruptive and aggressive behaviour in children and young people. This behaviour is persistent (lasting over 6 months), significantly violates age-appropriate expectations and is therefore in excess of normal childhood behaviour.[1] The WHO recognises subgroups of conduct disorder (more common in children aged 11–12 or older) and oppositional defiant disorder (ODD), which is predominantly a disorder of younger children.

Children with ODD display repeated defiant, disobedient and disruptive behaviours that go beyond mere 'naughtiness'.[1] However, the category of ODD does not include the more aggressive forms of behaviour, or delinquency.

Behaviours exhibited in conduct disorder are more extreme than in ODD. Examples given by the WHO[1] include: excessive levels of fighting or bullying, cruelty to other people or animals, severe destructiveness to property, fire setting, stealing, repeated lying, truancy from school and running away from home, unusually frequent and severe temper tantrums, and disobedience. For diagnosis of a conduct disorder, any of these behaviours should not be isolated antisocial acts but part of a persistent pattern. Conduct disorder can also be divided into socialised and unsocialised forms, depending on how well the child is integrated into his or her peer group.

Conduct disorders are the most common mental health disorder in children and young people[56] and are more common in boys than in girls. The 2004 Child Mental Health Survey of 5–16 year olds in Great Britain[57] reported a prevalence of 5.8% (7.5% in boys and 3.9% in girls). Prevalence increases with age, with 4.9% of children in the 5–10 age group meeting diagnostic criteria compared with 6.6% in the 11–16 age band. These disorders are more common in the lower socioeconomic groups, and among children looked after by local authorities – in the 2003 survey of the mental health of looked-after children, 36% were found to have a conduct disorder.[58]

Conduct disorders are associated with considerable co-morbidity. In the 2004 survey, 35% of children with conduct disorder had at least one other mental disorder, most commonly an emotional disorder or ADHD. The diagnosis has wide-ranging implications for the child's educational, social and health outcomes. It is associated with poor educational performance, tobacco, drug and alcohol misuse, and increased contact with the criminal justice system, as well as an increased risk of mental health disorders in adult life,[2] with a worse prognosis for earlier onset. Up to 50% may go on to develop antisocial personality disorder.[2]

1.8 Dementia

Dementia is a progressive deterioration in higher cognitive function to an extent that impairs daily activities. 'Higher cognitive function' implies brain functions such as memory, language, concentration and reasoning (as opposed to 'lower' functions such as those controlling movement, breathing or metabolism), so dementia is a 'syndrome' (ie a collection of symptoms) rather than a specific disease. There are many diseases that cause dementia, and dementia can occur at any age; however, the most common forms occur in old age and arise predominantly from Alzheimer's disease, vascular disorders and the presence of Lewy bodies. Alzheimer's disease is a specific disease characterised by loss of brain cells and particular abnormalities in the brain that can be seen under the microscope. It tends to affect memory function first with other brain functions being lost as the disease progresses. Vascular dementia describes a loss of brain function due to strokes or other disturbances of cerebral blood supply, and occurs independently from but often in association with Alzheimer's disease, particularly when dementia develops in late old age. Lewy body dementia is a more recently recognised entity characterised by particular abnormalities in brain tissue seen under the microscope; similar to vascular dementia, it also predominantly occurs in combination with other causes and overlaps with Parkinson's disease.

The prevalence of dementia is strongly related to age. A recent UK report estimated that 1% of people aged 65–69 were affected, rising to 33% of people aged 95 and over.[59] The incidence of dementia rises from around 1 per 1,000 per year of 65–69 year olds to 20 per 1,000 per year of 80–84 year olds.[60] It is still a matter of debate what happens to these figures in very advanced old age (eg above the age of 100), as some studies suggest a levelling off of risk whereas others suggest a continued increase. However, as a result of the association between dementia and increased age, and increased life expectancy in most populations in the world, dementia is becoming much more common. In 2007 it was estimated that there were around 680,000 people with dementia in the UK and that this figure would rise to 940,000 by 2021.[59] Dementia is a major cause of disability and places substantial economic costs on society, both because of the need for formal support services and institutional care in people with more advanced disease, and because of the often hidden costs for family members or other carers. The cost of dementia for the UK in 2007 was estimated to be £17bn per year, or £25,500 per person affected per year.[59]

Similar to many common chronic disorders, dementia has mixed genetic and environmental risk factors. Several genetic abnormalities have been found for the rare early onset dementias and one gene, apolipoprotein E, has been found to affect risk of the more common late-onset forms.[61] The main environmental risk factors are those that influence vascular risk, such as high blood pressure, diabetes, high cholesterol, obesity, lack of exercise, poor quality diet and smoking, all of which have been established to be risk factors not only for vascular dementia but also for Alzheimer's disease.[62] Dementia is also associated with lower levels of education, although the mechanism of this association is not clearly understood. Gender is not a risk factor for dementia but because of longer female longevity there tend to be more women with dementia in any given population. Other putative risk factors include head injury, heavy alcohol use and depression.

1.9 Mental health services

Most people with mental disorders in the UK who seek healthcare for their symptoms are treated in primary care,[63] although patients may present with symptoms such as fatigue and poor appetite that are not recognised as symptoms of an underlying mental disorder; as a result, as many as half of all cases of common mental disorder are undetected by the general practitioner (GP).[63] In the 2007 Adult Psychiatric Morbidity Survey, only a third of people with common mental disorders assessed as severe enough to require treatment had used a healthcare service for their emotional difficulties, most commonly their GP.[4] In primary care, common mental disorders may be treated by psychological therapy services, which usually offer cognitive–behavioural therapy, or medication such as antidepressants.

Severe cases and rarer illnesses in the UK tend to be referred to secondary care mental health services – in 2010–11, 2.8% of adults in England used hospital or community mental health services.[64] Mental health services are based predominantly in the community, in multidisciplinary community mental health teams. Such teams usually include a consultant psychiatrist, psychiatric nurses, a psychologist and social workers. There are also specialised teams in the community, eg crisis resolution teams that focus on intensive home treatment to avoid hospitalisation, early intervention teams for young people presenting with psychotic symptoms, rehabilitation teams, and assertive outreach teams for people with severe and chronic disorders (usually psychotic disorders) who need care but are reluctant to engage with services. Inpatient services are used predominantly for acute presentations that cannot be managed in the community, and patients with chronic severe illness are typically now cared for in supported accommodation rather than the large asylums of the past. The overall provision of NHS acute psychiatric beds for adults and elderly people is 4.3 per 10,000 of the total population,[65] with provision for people aged over 65 roughly double that for working age adults in relation to their population numbers.

1.10 Summary

> - Mental disorders comprise a spectrum of conditions ranging from the mild and transient to the severe and disabling.
> - Mental disorders are common, occurring to some degree in about a quarter of adults and in around 10% of children and adolescents in any year.
> - Most people with mental disorders are cared for in the community, predominantly by GPs, but also by specialist multidisciplinary teams. A minority of people with mental disorders are managed in secondary care inpatient facilities.
> - Mental disorders are associated with increased rates of a range of health risk behaviours (such as smoking, alcohol and drug misuse, poor diet, less physical activity, self-harm), poor educational and employment outcomes, homelessness, social stigmatisation, marginalisation, and reduced uptake or delivery of health services, including for health risk behaviour and physical illness.
> - Life expectancy among people with many mental disorders is substantially lower than that of the general population.

References

1 World Health Organization. *The ICD-10 Classification of Mental and Behavioural Disorders. Diagnostic criteria for research.* Geneva: WHO, 1992.

2 Van Os J, Kapur S. Schizophrenia. *The Lancet* 2009;374:635–45.

3 American Psychiatric Association. *Diagnostic and Statistical Manual of Mental Disorders,* 4th edn (DSM-IV). Washington DC: American Psychiatric Association, 2000.

4 McManus S, Meltzer H, Brugha T, Bebbington P, Jenkins R. Adult Psychiatric Morbidity Survey 2007. Results of a household survey. The NHS Health & Social Care Information Centre, Social Care Statistics, 2009. www.ic.nhs.uk/pubs/

5 Kirkbride J, Errazuriz A, Croudace T, *et al.* Incidence of schizophrenia and other psychoses in England, 1950–2009: A systematic review and meta analyses. *PLoS One* 2012;7(3).

6 Department of Health. *Safety First: Five-year report of the National Confidential Inquiry into Suicide and Homicide by People with Mental Illness.* London: Department of Health, 2001.

7 Thornicroft G. *Shunned: Discrimination against people with mental illness.* Oxford: Oxford University Press, 2006.

8 Thornicroft G, Brohan E, Rose D, Sartorius N, Leese M, INDIGO Study Group. Global pattern of experienced and anticipated discrimination against people with schizophrenia: a cross-sectional survey. *The Lancet* 2009;31:408–15.

9 Howard LM, Barley EA, Davies E, *et al.* Cancer diagnosis in people with severe mental illness: practical and ethical issues. *Lancet Oncology* 2010;11:797–804.

10 Lorant V, Deliège D, Eaton W, *et al.* Socioeconomic inequalities in depression: a meta-analysis. *American Journal of Epidemiology* 2003;157:98–112.

11 Muntaner C, Eaton WW, Miech R, O'Campo P. Socioeconomic position and major mental disorders. *Epidemiological Reviews* 2004;26:53–62.

12 Chang CK, Hayes RD, Perera G, *et al*. Life expectancy at birth for people with serious mental illness and other major disorders from a secondary mental health care case register in London. *PLoS One* 2011;6(5).

13 Osborn DP, Levy G, Nazareth I, *et al*. Relative risk of cardiovascular and cancer mortality in people with severe mental illness from the United Kingdom's General Practice Research Database. *Archives of General Psychiatry* 2007;64:242–9.

14 Hennekens CH, Hennekens AR, Hollar D, Casey DE. Schizophrenia and increased risks of cardiovascular disease. *American Heart Journal* 2005;150:1115–21.

15 Aubin HJ, Rollema H, Svensson TH, Winterer G. Smoking, quitting, and psychiatric disease: a review. *Neuroscience and Biobehavioral Reviews* 2012;36:271–84.

16 King M, Walker C, Levy G, *et al*. Development and validation of an international risk prediction algorithm for episodes of major depression in general practice attendees: the PredictD study. *Archives of General Psychiatry* 2008;65:1368–76.

17 Nanni V, Uher R, Danese A. Childhood maltreatment predicts unfavourable course of illness and treatment outcome in depression: A meta-analysis. *American Journal of Psychiatry* 2012;169:141–51.

18 Trevillion K, Oram S, Feder G, Howard LM. Experiences of domestic violence and mental disorders: a systematic review and meta-analysis. King's College London, 2012.

19 Tyrer P, Seivewright H, Johnson T. The Nottingham Study of Neurotic Disorder: predictors of 12-year outcome of dysthymic, panic and generalized anxiety disorder. *Psychological Medicine* 2004;34:1385–94.

20 Horwath E, Weissman MM. The epidemiology and cross-national presentation of obsessive–compulsive disorder. *Psychiatric Clinics of North America* 2000;23:493–507

21 Skoog G, Skoog I. 40-year follow-up of patients with obsessive-compulsive disorder. *Archives of General Psychiatry* 1999;56:121–7.

22 Stewart S, Geller D, Jenike M, *et al*. Long-term outcome of pediatric obsessive–compulsive disorder: a meta-analysis and qualitative review of the literature. *Acta Psychiatrica Scandinavica* 2004;110:4–13.

23 National Institute for Health and Clinical Excellence – The British Psychological Society and The Royal College of Psychiatrists. *NICE CG31 Obsessive compulsive disorder: Core interventions in the treatment of obsessive compulsive disorder*. London: NICE, 2006.

24 Brewin CR, Andrews B, Valentine JD. Meta-analysis of risk factors for posttraumatic stress disorder in trauma-exposed adults. *Journal of Consulting Clinical Psychology* 2000;68:748–66.

25 Ozer EJ, Best SR, Lipsey TL, Weiss DS. Predictors of posttraumatic stress disorder and symptoms in adults: a meta-analysis. *Psychological Bulletin* 2003;129:52–73.

26 Treasure J, Claudino AM, Zucker N. Eating disorders. *The Lancet* 2010;375:583–93.

27 Berkman ND, Lohr KN, Bulik CM. Outcomes of eating disorders: a systematic review of the literature. *International Journal of Eating Disorders* 2007;40:293–309.

28 Keel PK, Mitchell JE, Miller KB, Davis TL, Crow SJ. Long-term outcome of bulimia nervosa. *Archives of General Psychiatry* 1999;56:63–9.

29 Jacobi C, Hayward C, de Zwaan M, Kraemer HC, Agras WS. Coming to terms with risk factors for eating disorders: application of risk terminology and suggestions for a general taxonomy. *Psychological Bulletin* 2004;130:19–65.

30 Jacobi C, Fittig E, Bryson SW, *et al*. Who is really at risk? Identifying risk factors for subthreshold and full syndrome eating disorders in a high-risk sample. *Psychological Medicine* 2011;41:1939–49.

31 Wessely S, Nimnuan C, Sharpe M. Functional somatic syndromes:one or many? *The Lancet* 1999;354:936–39.

32 Ring A, Dowrick CF, Humphris GM, Davies J, Salmon P. The somatising effect of clinical consultation: what patients and doctors say and do not say when patients present medically unexplained physical symptoms. *Social Science and Medicine* 2005;61:1505–15.

33 Nimnuan C, Hotopf M, Wessely S. Medically unexplained symptoms: an epidemiological study in seven specialities. *Journal of Psychosomatic Research* 2001;31:361–7.

34 Warwick HMC, Clark DM, Cobb AM, Salkovskis PM. A controlled trial of cognitive behavioural treatment of hypochondriasis. *British Journal of Psychiatry* 1996;169:189–85.

35 Escobar JI, Manu P, Matthews D, *et al*. Medically unexplained physical symptoms, somatization disorder and abridged somatization: studies with the Diagnostic Interview Schedule. *Psychiatric Developments* 1989;3:235–45.

36 Hotopf M, Mayou R, Wadsworth M, Wessely S. Childhood risk factors for adult medically unexplained symptoms: results of a national birth cohort study. *American Journal of Psychiatry* 1999;156:1796–800.

37 Smith GR. Course of somatization and its effects on utilization of health care resources. *Psychosomatics* 1994;35:263–67.

38 McGrath J, Saha S, Chant D, Welham J. Schizophrenia: a concise overview of incidence, prevalence, and mortality. *Epidemiological Reviews* 2008;30:67–76.

39 Merikangas KR, Akiskal HS, Angst J, *et al*. Lifetime and 12-month prevalence of bipolar spectrum disorder in the National Comorbidity Survey replication. *Archives of General Psychiatry* 2007;64:543–52.

40 Müller-Oerlinghausen B, Berghöfer A, Bauer M. Bipolar disorder. *The Lancet* 2002;359:241–7.

41 Craddock N, Jones I. Molecular genetics of bipolar disorder. *British Journal of Psychiatry* 2001;178:S128–33.

42 Lloyd T, Kennedy N, Fearon P, *et al*. Incidence of bipolar affective disorder in three UK cities: results from the AESOP study. *British Journal of Psychiatry* 2005;186:126–31.

43 Daruy-Filho L, Brietzke E, Lafer B, Grassi-Oliveira R. Childhood maltreatment and clinical outcomes of bipolar disorder. *Acta Psychiatrica Scandinavica* 2011;124:427–34.

44 Coid J, Yang M, Tyrer P, Roberts A, Ullrich S. Prevalence and correlates of personality disorder in Great Britain. *British Journal of Psychiatry* 2006;188:423–31

45 Kendall T, Pilling ST, Tyrer P, *et al*. Guideline Development Groups. Borderline and antisocial personality disorders: summary of NICE guidance. *British Medical Journal* 2009;338:b93.

46 Samuels J. Personality disorders: Epidemiology and public health issues. *International Review of Psychiatry* 2011;23:223–33.

47 Dixon-Gordon KL, Turner BJ, Chapman AL. Psychotherapy for personality disorders. *International Review of Psychiatry* 2011;23:282–302.

48 Ford T, Goodman R, Meltzer H. The British Child and Adolescent Mental Health Survey 1999: the prevalence of DSM-IV disorders. *Journal of the American Academy of Child and Adolescent Psychiatry* 2003;42:1203–11.

49 National Institute for Health and Clinical Excellence – The British Psychological Society and The Royal College of Psychiatrists. *CG72 Attention deficit hyperactivity disorder: Diagnosis and management of ADHD in children, young people and adults*. London: NICE, 2009.

50 Faraone S, Biederman J, Mick E. The age-dependent decline of attention deficit hyperactivity disorder: a meta-analysis of follow-up studies. *Psychological Medicine* 2006;36:159–65

51 Simon V, Czobor P, Bálint S, Mészáros Á, Bitter I. Prevalence and correlates of adult attention-deficit hyperactivity disorder: meta-analysis. *British Journal of Psychiatry* 2009;194:204–11.

52 Young S, Toone B. Comorbidity and psychosocial profile of adults with attention deficit hyperactivity disorder. *Personality and Individual Differences* 2003;35:743–55.

53 Biederman J, Petty CR, Fried R, *et al*. Educational and occupational underachievement in adults with ADHD: a controlled study. *Journal of Clinical Psychiatry* 2008;69:1271–22.

54 Thapar A, Cooper M, Jefferies R, Stergiakouli E. What causes attention deficit hyperactivity disorder? *Archives of Disease in Childhood* 2012;97:260–5.

55 McCann D, Barrett A, Cooper A, *et al*. Food additives and hyperactive behaviour in 3-year-old and 8/9-year-old children in the community: a randomised, double-blind, placebo-controlled trial. *The Lancet* 2007;3:1560–67.

56 National Institute for Health and Clinical Excellence and Social Care Institute for Excellence. *Conduct disorders in children and young people: draft scope for consultation*. London: NICE, 2011.

57 Green H, McGinnity A, Meltzer H, Ford T, Goodman R. *Mental health of children and young people in Great Britain, 2004*. Newport: Office for National Statistics, 2005.

58 Meltzer H CT, Gatward R, Goodman R, Ford T. *The mental health of young people looked after by local authorities in England*. Newport: Office for National Statistics, 2003.

59 Knapp M, Prince M, Albanesem E, *et al*. *Dementia UK*. London: Alzheimer's Society, 2007.

60 Ott A, Slooter A, Hofman A, *et al*. Smoking and the risk of dementia and Alzheimer's disease in a population-based cohort study: the Rotterdam Study. In: Ott A (ed.), *Risk of dementia*. Delft: Judels en Brinkman BV, 1997: 89–98.

61 Verghese PB, Castellano JM, Holtzman DM. Apolipoprotein E in Alzheimer's disease and other neurological disorders. *The Lancet Neurology* 2011;10:241–52.

62 Stewart R. Cardiovascular factors in Alzheimer's disease. *Journal of Neurology, Neurosurgery, and Psychiatry* 1998;65:143–7.

63 Goldberg DP, Huxley P. *Common mental disorders: a bio-social model*. London: Tavistock, 1992.

64 NHS Information Centre. www.ic.nhs.uk/article/2021/Website-Search?productid=2567&q=Fifth+report+from+Mental+Health+Minimum+Data+Set+%28MHMDS%29&sort=Relevance&size=10&page=1&area=both#top [Accessed 1 July 2012]

65 Glover G. Adult mental health care in England. *European Archives of Psychiatry Clinical Neuroscience* 2007;257:71–82.

2 | Smoking among people with mental disorders

2.1 Introduction

There is long-standing evidence from British[1] and international[2] studies that smoking prevalence is substantially higher among people with mental disorders than in the general population. The strength of this association tends to increase with increasing severity of mental disorder, and the highest prevalence of smoking is found among psychiatric inpatients.[1,3] To date, evidence on this association in UK populations has been limited primarily to that available from the Adult Psychiatric Morbidity Surveys (APMS) carried out by the NHS Information Centre. In this chapter we summarise findings from the APMS, and explore data from alternative sources, to assess trends in smoking, cessation behaviour and support, and other characteristics of smoking in more detail among adults with mental disorders in the UK.

2.2 Data and methods

This chapter draws on three sources of data: the Health Survey for England[4] (HSE) and the APMS,[5] which are both national surveys of the English population, and The Health Improvement Network[6] (THIN), a database containing the primary care medical records of over 8 million patients registered with general practitioners (GPs) throughout the UK.

2.2.1 Health Survey for England

The HSE is a cross-sectional survey that has questioned samples of adults aged 16 and over every year since 1993. The most recent data available at the time of writing are from the 2010 survey, in which responses on smoking were obtained from 8,369 participants. The survey included three measures of mental health:

1 Participants were asked: 'Do you have any longstanding illness, disability or infirmity? By longstanding I mean anything that has troubled you over a

period of time, or that is likely to affect you over a period of time?'. Answers are categorised into illness groups, from which people who reported longstanding mental illness, depression or anxiety can be identified.
2. Participants were asked for the names of prescribed medications that they had taken within the 7 days before being interviewed, and answers can be used to identify those taking psychoactive medications including antipsychotics, antimanics, antidepressants and anxiolytics.
3. Participants were asked to complete the 12-item General Health Questionnaire (GHQ-12),[7] which screens for non-psychotic psychiatric disorders by assessing attributes including current ability to concentrate, ability to make decisions and self-belief in short-term relation to their usual state. A score of 3 or more out of 12 is taken here to indicate the probable presence of a non-psychotic psychiatric disorder.

Several measures of smoking behaviour are available from the HSE. Current smokers are defined as those who respond positively to the question 'Do you smoke cigarettes at all nowadays?'. Ex-regular smokers are identified as those who report having once smoked at least one cigarette a day, but are no longer smoking. From these measures of current and ex-smoking a quit ratio of the proportion of ever smokers who have quit can be calculated.

All current smokers are asked whether they would like to give up smoking altogether, how difficult they would find it to go without smoking for a whole day, how long after waking they smoke their first cigarette of the day and how many cigarettes they consume daily. The Heaviness of Smoking Index (HSI) can be calculated from these last two indicators to illustrate a smoker's strength of addiction to cigarettes.[8] An HSI score of 5 or 6 (out of a maximum of 6) is taken here to indicate heavy addiction.

2.2.2 Adult Psychiatric Morbidity Survey

The APMS is designed to describe and quantify the occurrence and extent of psychiatric problems, associated disabilities and service use in England. At the time of writing the most recent available data are from 2007, when 7,393 adults living in private households in England were surveyed. Data are also available from household surveys carried out in 2000 and 1993.

Smokers are identified in the APMS using the same questions as in the HSE, although the APMS excludes the small number of self-reported current smokers who report smoking an average of fewer than seven cigarettes per week. The APMS does not identify ex-regular smokers, only those who have ever tried a cigarette, and so quit ratios equivalent to those in the HSE cannot be calculated. However, the HSI can be calculated for current smokers in the same way as in the HSE.

The APMS uses several established and validated tools to identify patients with mental disorders.[9] The revised Clinical Interview Schedule[10] (CIS-R) was used to assess patients for the presence within the last week of several common mental disorders, including depressive episodes, phobias, generalised anxiety disorder, obsessive–compulsive disorder, panic disorder, and mixed anxiety and depression. A total CIS-R score of 12 or more is taken here to indicate the presence of a common mental disorder. The Trauma Screening Questionnaire[11] (TSQ) was used to screen participants for post-traumatic stress disorder (PTSD) within the last 2 weeks, the Adult Self-Report Scale–v1.1[12] (ASRS) assessed people for attention deficit hyperactivity disorder (ADHD) within the last 6 months and the SCOFF eating disorders questionnaire[13] assessed for an eating disorder within the last year. A subsample of participants was also screened by clinically trained interviewers to detect probable psychosis.[9] The label of 'any mental disorder' is used here to identify participants with at least one of the common mental disorders listed above, PTSD, ADHD, an eating disorder or probable psychosis.

Several self-reported measures of mental health are also available in APMS data, including whether participants have made one or more suicide attempts in the last year, whether they have spoken to their GP in the past year about a mental, nervous or emotional problem, and whether they are currently receiving counselling or using a psychoactive medication for a mental, nervous or emotional problem.

In relation to the objectives of this report, APMS and HSE data share three main limitations: first, their sample sizes are such that estimates of smoking prevalence within demographic or mental health subgroups are often based on small numbers and hence imprecise; second, the reliance on self-reported measures of mental health and smoking behaviour introduces the possibility of biased estimates of these outcomes; and, third, that as household surveys both the APMS and HSE exclude groups of people known to have higher rates of mental illness and a higher smoking prevalence, including those living in mental healthcare institutions, prisons and temporary housing, and homeless individuals. Both surveys are therefore likely to underestimate the true population prevalence of mental illness and smoking. However, as a supplement to the first household psychiatric morbidity survey, in 1994 a survey of 1,200 adults living in institutions specifically catering for people with mental illness[14] was carried out, as well as a survey of 1,100 adult homeless people (living in hostels or similar institutions or sleeping rough and using day centres).[15] In 1997, 3,500 prisoners in England and Wales were similarly surveyed.[16] At the end of this chapter we present headline findings from these surveys, with the caveat that the data are now over 15 years old (further data on smoking prevalence among homeless people and prisoner populations are presented in Chapter 7).

2.2.3 The Health Improvement Network

THIN is a dataset of electronic primary care medical records, established in 2003 by EPIC[6] licence holders of a historical part of the General Practice Research Database (GPRD). General practices using the Vision[17] electronic practice management software can choose to contribute their data to THIN, and data from contributing practices are uploaded electronically on a monthly basis. Ethics approval for the collection and use of these data has been granted by the NHS South-East Multicentre Research Ethics Committee. By September 2010, THIN contained records for almost 8 million patients from 495 practices throughout the UK; these patients are broadly representative of the UK population in terms of their age, sex, medical conditions and death rates.[18] THIN contains details of consultations with members of the primary healthcare team, investigation results, prescribed medications and lifestyle information such as smoking behaviour. Information is recorded using Read codes, a hierarchical dictionary of medical terminology.[19]

The data used in this chapter are derived from 2,493,085 patients aged 16 and over who were registered with a THIN practice for the year from 1 July 2009 to 30 June 2010. Patients with mental disorders were identified in two ways: Read codes were used to identify those with a record of one or more of several specified mental disorders during the study period, corresponding to ICD-10 categories (Box 2.1), and *British National Formulary* (BNF) codes[20] were used to identify patients who had been prescribed a psychoactive medication (antipsychotic, antimanic, antidepressant or anxiolytic) during the study period.

Patients who smoked during the study period were identified as those with a relevant smoking-related Read code recorded in their medical records during the study year. Patients were also classified as smokers if their smoking status was not recorded during the study period, but their last-recorded status before the start

Box 2.1 ICD-10 codes for mental disorders identified in THIN patients

F20–F29	Schizophrenia, schizotypal and delusional disorders
F31	Bipolar affective disorder
F32–F33	Depression
F40–F48	Neurotic, stress-related and somatoform disorders
F50	Eating disorders
F60	Specific personality disorders
F90	Hyperkinetic disorders, including ADHD

ADHD, attention deficit hyperactivity disorder; ICD-10, *International Classification of Diseases*, 10th revision; THIN, The Health Improvement Network.

of the study indicated that they were smoking. This method has been shown to provide smoking prevalence estimates closely similar to national survey data.[18] We also used Read codes to identify patients whose notes contained a record of cessation advice having been delivered in the year to mid-2010, and BNF codes to identify patients prescribed one of the three smoking cessation medications (nicotine replacement therapy (NRT), bupropion and varenicline) in the study period.

The major strength of the THIN dataset for this analysis is the large sample size and hence relatively high precision of estimates of smoking in relation to mental disorder. However, THIN data also have limitations. Not all patients with mental health conditions will be managed solely in the primary care setting, because those with diagnoses such as schizophrenia or bipolar disorder are also likely to be managed by specialist teams in secondary care. Details of treatments or diagnoses delivered to these patients in inpatient or outpatient secondary care settings are not necessarily entered into the primary care medical record. As a result, analyses using THIN data may underestimate the number of patients with mental health conditions. Conversely, many medications prescribed for mental disorders may also be used for other indications, such as anxiolytics as sleeping tablets, or antidepressants for relief of chronic pain, thus leading to potential overestimation of the proportion of patients receiving medication for mental disorder.

Since the introduction of the Quality and Outcomes Framework (QOF) in 2004, GPs have received financial incentives to record and update patients' smoking status. This has resulted in convergence, since 2006, of smoking prevalence estimates from THIN and those derived from representative national surveys, although there remains a shortfall in the recorded prevalence in some groups of patients, particularly young men.[18] Ex-smoking is less well recorded, so quit ratios cannot be calculated from THIN data with confidence. The QOF also incentivised GPs to document their delivery of cessation advice to smokers with particular chronic diseases, including schizophrenia, bipolar disorder and other psychoses, but, although rates of recording of advice increased as a result of this initiative, there is evidence that this documentation might not accurately represent advice given, remembered by the patient or acted upon.[21] Similarly, although rates of prescribing of smoking cessation medications in THIN are similar to levels of pharmacy dispensing,[22] a record of a medication being prescribed to a patient does not mean that medication was used as indicated or resulted in a successful quit attempt, and does not capture patients who purchase NRT over the counter.

The relevant features of the three data sources used in this chapter are summarised in Table 2.1.

Table 2.1 Description of data sources used in this chapter

	HSE	APMS	THIN
Year of survey	2010	2007	2009–10
Sample size	8,369	7,393	2,493,085
Geographical coverage	England	England	UK
Outcome measures reported			
Smoking prevalence			
By self-reported longstanding mental health	✔		
By specific diagnoses		✔	✔
By prescription of psychoactive medications	✔	✔	✔
By GHQ-12	✔		
By CIS-R		✔	
By self-reported mental health service use		✔	
By self-reported suicide attempt		✔	
Quit ratio	✔		
Heaviness of Smoking Index	✔	✔	
Daily cigarette consumption	✔	✔	
Smokers reporting wanting to quit	✔		
Smokers reporting quitting would be difficult	✔		
Smokers receiving cessation advice			✔
Smokers receiving cessation medication prescription			✔

APMS, Adult Psychiatric Morbidity Survey; CIS-R, revised Clinical Interview Schedule; GHQ-12, 12-item General Health Questionnaire; HSE. Health Survey for England; THIN, The Health Improvement Network.

2.3 Smoking prevalence

2.3.1 HSE

In 2010, HSE data estimate the prevalence of smoking among adults in England to be 20%, a figure almost identical to that estimated for the same year in the much larger General Lifestyle Survey of Great Britain.[23] However, smoking prevalence was significantly higher in those reporting indicators of mental disorder (Table 2.2). Among the 4% of HSE participants reporting longstanding anxiety, depression or another mental health issue, 37% were smokers, a significantly higher proportion than in participants not reporting these conditions. After taking into account differences in age, sex and social class, HSE data suggest that participants with a longstanding mental health condition are twice as likely to be smokers compared with those without (odds ratio (OR) = 2.2, 95% confidence interval (CI) 1.7–2.8). Smoking prevalence was also significantly higher, at 27%, among the 19% of HSE participants who scored 3 or

Table 2.2 Smoking prevalence according to mental health diagnosis and medication use (HSE, 2010[4])

	Number[a]	Prevalence of diagnosis[b] (95% CI)	Smoking prevalence (95% CI)
All participants	8,369		20.1 (18.9–21.3)
Reports current non-psychotic psychiatric morbidity (GHQ-12 3+)	1,440	19.3 (18.2–20.4)	27.3 (24.7–30.0)
Reports a longstanding mental health condition	353	4.11 (3.57–4.73)	37.4 (31.9–43.1)
Reports taking a psychoactive medication in the last 7 days	491	5.21 (4.72–5.74)	27.0 (22.4–31.5)
Antipsychotic	30	0.36 (0.24–0.54)	44.7 (26.7–64.7)
Antimanic	16	0.17 (0.00–0.29)	49.5 (26.3–72.8)
Antidepressant	468	4.93 (4.45–5.47)	26.6 (22.3–31.2)
Anxiolytic	25	0.26 (0.18–0.39)	41.0 (22.3–62.8)

[a]Unweighted.
[b]Weighted to account for survey design.
CI, confidence interval; GHQ-12, 12-item General Health Questionnaire; HSE, Health Survey for England.

more on the GHQ-12, and was also 27% among the 5% of participants who reported having taken a psychoactive medication within the past 7 days.

As Fig 2.1 shows, data from earlier waves of the HSE demonstrate a sustained and progressive decline in smoking prevalence over the past two decades among participants not reporting a longstanding mental health condition, whereas rates among those reporting these conditions have remained almost unchanged during this period. Although a drop to 37% was observed in the most recent, 2010, survey, further surveys are needed to confirm whether this is the start of a downward trend.

2.3.2 APMS

Similar findings of higher smoking prevalence among those with a diagnosed mental disorder or using psychoactive medication are evident in the 2007 APMS data (Table 2.3). Smoking prevalence within specific diagnostic groups ranged from 25% (eating disorders) to 56% (probable psychosis) and, among those with a common mental disorder, defined as a score of 12 or more on the CIS-R, 34%

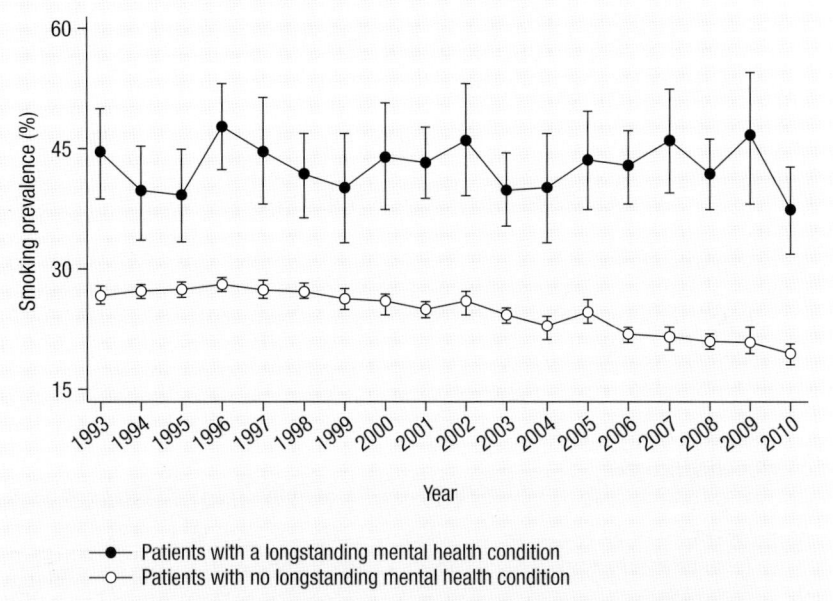

Fig 2.1 Changes in smoking prevalence between 1993 and 2010 in participants with or without longstanding mental health conditions (with 95% confidence intervals (CIs); data from the Health Survey for England (HSE)).

were smokers. Of the 11% of adults in England estimated by APMS to have consulted a GP in the past year for a mental, nervous or emotional complaint, 33% were smokers, of the 3% of adults who had received counselling for a mental, nervous or emotional complaint at the time of the survey, 35% were smokers, and of the 0.7% of adults who had made one or more suicide attempts in the last year, 57% were smokers.

2.3.3 THIN

Data from the THIN primary care database add further confirmation of the high prevalence of smoking among those with diagnosed mental disorders and those taking psychoactive medications (Table 2.4). Although there is inevitable inconsistency between the proportions in disease-specific diagnostic groups and those using related medications (eg those with diagnosed depression and those taking antidepressants), which probably reflects both a failure to regularly update diagnostic recording and the use of psychoactive drugs for other indications (see section 2.2.3), smoking prevalence in all the groups in Table 2.3 is substantially and statistically significantly higher than in the population without these morbidities or prescription drug use.

Table 2.3 Smoking prevalence according to mental health diagnosis and medication use (APMS, 2007[9])

	Number[a]	Prevalence (%) of diagnosis[b] (95% CI)	Smoking prevalence (%)[g] (95% CI)
All participants	7,393		22.2 (21.0–23.4)
Reporting a common mental disorder (CIS-R 12+)[c]	1,185	15.1 (14.1–16.0)	34.0 (31.0–37.1)
Reporting any mental health disorder	1,382	17.8 (16.8–18.9)	33.0 (30.2–35.8)
Depressive episode[c]	255	2.98 (2.60–3.42)	39.8 (33.2–46.8)
Phobias[c]	160	2.03 (1.71–2.41)	42.8 (34.0–50.1)
Generalised anxiety disorder[c]	363	4.39 (3.92–4.91)	37.4 (31.9–43.4)
Obsessive–compulsive disorder[c]	86	1.11 (0.85–1.44)	40.2 (28.3–53.5)
Panic disorder[c]	83	1.13 (0.89–1.43)	28.9 (19.6–40.4)
Mixed anxiety and depression[c]	639	8.39 (7.66–9.18)	31.1 (27.1–35.3)
Probable psychosis[f]	29	0.39 (0.25–0.60)	56.0 (33.3–76.3)
Post-traumatic stress disorder[d]	215	2.89 (2.50–3.34)	40.4 (33.1–48.2)
Attention deficit hyper-activity disorder[e]	39	0.57 (0.41–0.79)	39.1 (23.4–57.5)
Eating disorder[f]	108	1.55 (1.26–1.92)	25.3 (17.3–35.4)
Currently taking a psychoactive medication	501	5.65 (5.14–6.21)	35.0 (30.3–39.9)
Antipsychotic	40	0.47 (0.32–0.70)	59.2 (41.3–75.0)
Antimanic	12	0.14 (0.08–0.24)	8.86 (1.59–36.9)
Antidepressant	417	4.69 (4.23–5.21)	33.8 (28.9–39.1)
Anxiolytic	79	0.85 (0.67–1.07)	41.6 (30.0–54.3)

[a]Unweighted.
[b]Weighted to account for survey design.
[c]In the past week.
[d]In the past 2 weeks.
[e]In the past 6 months.
[f]In the past year.
[g]Unadjusted for age (hence any difference from published APMS figures[9]).
APMS, Adult Psychiatric Morbidity Survey; CI, confidence interval; CIS-R, revised Clinical Interview Schedule.

Table 2.4 Smoking prevalence according to psychiatric diagnosis and medication use in the past year (THIN data, 2009–10[6])

	Number	Prevalence (%) of diagnosis (95% CI)	Smoking prevalence (%) (95% CI)
All patients	2,493,085		19.7 (19.1–20.2)
Patients with one or more mental health diagnoses	106,108	4.26 (4.03–4.48)	30.3 (29.4–31.2)
Schizophrenia, schizotypal and delusional disorders	1,548	0.06 (0.06–0.07)	44.6 (41.4–47.7)
Bipolar affective disorder	1,084	0.04 (0.04–0.05)	36.7 (33.6–39.8)
Depression	62,841	2.52 (2.34–2.70)	31.4 (30.4–32.5)
Neurotic, stress-related and somatoform disorders	47,464	1.90 (1.76–2.05)	28.9 (27.8–29.9)
Eating disorders	1,055	0.04 (0.04–0.05)	23.1 (20.6–25.7)
Specific personality disorders	683	0.03 (0.02–0.03)	47.1 (43.0–51.3)
Hyperkinetic disorders, including ADHD	276	0.01 (0.01–0.01)	27.2 (21.0–33.3)
Patients prescribed one or more psychoactive medications	355,410	14.3 (14.0–14.6)	27.1 (26.3–27.9)
Antipsychotic	27,561	1.11 (1.06–1.15)	34.4 (33.2–35.6)
Lithium (antimanic)	3,502	0.14 (0.13–0.15)	30.2 (28.5–32.0)
Antidepressant	301,978	12.1 (11.8–12.4)	27.2 (26.4–28.0)
Anxiolytic	81,504	3.27 (3.14–3.40)	29.5 (28.5–30.5)

ADHD, attention deficit hyperactivity disorder; CI, confidence interval; THIN, The Health Improvement Network.

2.4 Population estimates

By combining the mid-2010 population estimates published by the Office for National Statistics[24] with our measures of the population prevalence of mental disorders and smoking within diagnostic groups, we have derived estimates of the number of people with a mental disorder in the UK, and the numbers that are smokers. Data (that do not allow for multiple diagnoses in the same person and hence are likely to be slight overestimates) are shown in Table 2.5, which

Table 2.5 Estimates of the number of adults in the UK with mental disorders, and numbers of those who smoke

	Estimated number in adult UK population	Estimated number of adult smokers
HSE (2010)[a]		
Reports current non-psychotic psychiatric morbidity (GHQ-12 3+)	9,761,026	2,663,784
Reports a longstanding mental health condition	2,081,879	777,790
Taken a psychoactive medication in the last 7 days	2,816,362	756,193
APMS (2007)[a]		
Reports a common mental disorder (CIS-R 12+)	7,648,754	2,600,576
Reports any mental disorder	9,016,412	2,975,416
Currently taking a psychoactive medication	2,861,951	1,001,683
THIN (2009–10)		
Diagnosed with one or more mental disorders in the last year	2,157,860	653,832
Prescribed psychoactive medication in the past year	7,243,522	1,962,994

[a]HSE and APMS data were collected in England only, though here prevalence figures for mental disorder and smoking have been applied to the UK total population estimate. APMS, Adult Psychiatric Morbidity Survey; CIS-R, revised Clinical Interview Schedule; GHQ-12, 12-item General Health Questionnaire; HSE, Health Survey for England; THIN, The Health Improvement Network.

demonstrates that, subject to the potential sources of error outlined above, there are approximately 2.6 million people in the UK with a common mental disorder who smoke (based on either the GHQ-12 or the CIS-R), and up to 3 million smokers with any mental disorder (based on data from the APMS). HSE data suggest that there are about 780,000 smokers with longstanding mental disorders in the UK, and 760,000 smokers who have recently taken a psychoactive medication; the higher smoking prevalence among those reporting psychoactive drug use in the APMS results in a higher estimate of approximately 1 million UK smokers currently taking such medication.

THIN data estimate a total of around 650,000 smokers with a record of mental disorder, and 2 million prescribed one or more psychoactive medications in the past year. As approximate estimates, the figures in Table 2.5 therefore demonstrate that up to 3 million, or 30% of the approximately 10 million smokers in the UK,[25] have evidence of mental disorder, and that in up to a million people, or 10% of all smokers, this mental disorder is longstanding and/or currently being treated with a psychoactive medication.

2.5 Variations in smoking prevalence among those with mental disorder by age, sex and socioeconomic status

HSE data broken down by age, sex and Index of Multiple Deprivation score[26] demonstrate that similar differences in smoking prevalence between subgroups are seen in participants who do and do not report a longstanding mental health condition. Smoking prevalence is higher in men, younger adults and those in the more deprived groups (Fig 2.2).

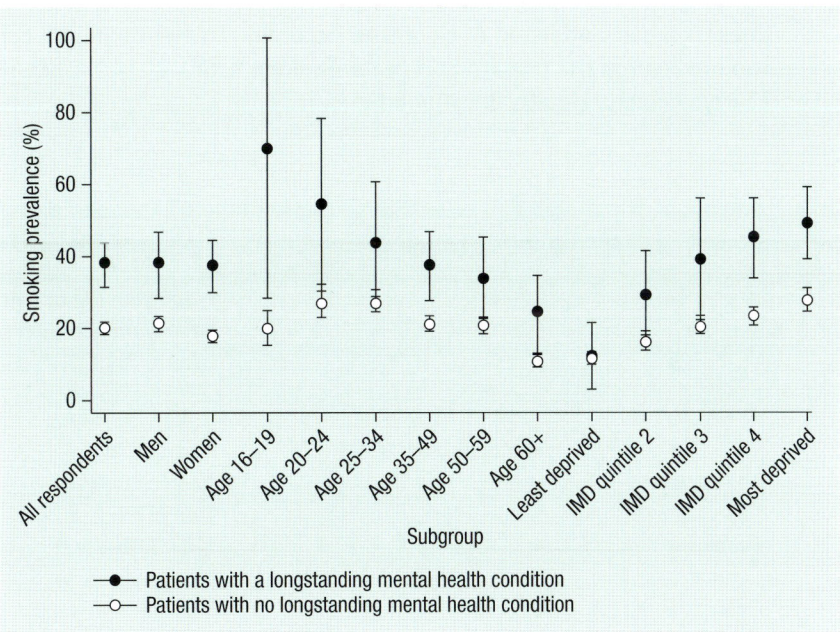

Fig 2.2 Differences in smoking prevalence between those with and those without a longstanding mental health condition according to age, sex and Index of Multiple Deprivation (IDM) score (Health Survey for England (HSE), 2010[4]).

2.6 Strength of addiction

Smokers with mental disorders are more heavily addicted to cigarettes than smokers in general. Among all smokers in the HSE, 5% were classified as heavily addicted according to the HSI; however, among those who scored 3 or more on

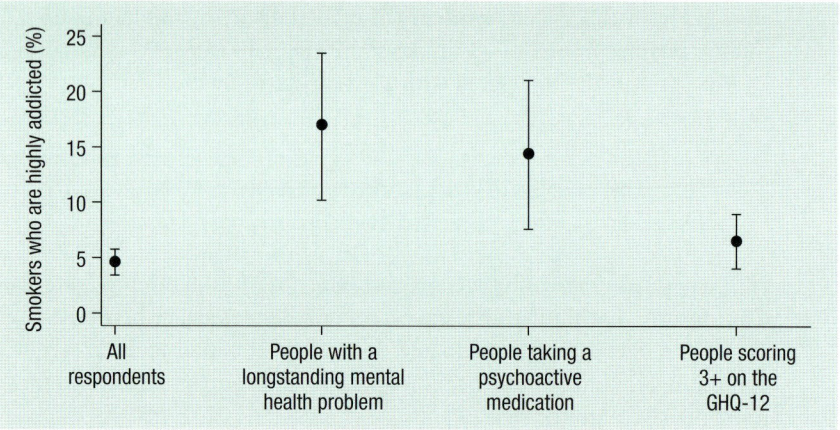

Fig 2.3 Estimated proportions (with 95% confidence intervals (CIs)) of smokers heavily addicted to cigarettes according to mental health condition and medication use (Health Survey for England (HSE), 2010[4]). GHQ-12, 12-item General Health Questionnaire.

Table 2.6 The proportion of smokers heavily addicted to cigarettes according to mental health diagnosis and medication use (APMS, 2007[9])

	Proportion (%) of smokers heavily addicted on HSI criteria (95% CI)[a]
All smokers	5.32 (4.26–6.64)
Reporting a common mental disorder (CIS-R 12+)	10.8 (7.87–14.6)
Any disorder	10.4 (7.70–13.8)
Depressive episode	14.9 (8.99–23.6)
Phobias	14.2 (7.16–26.2)
Generalised anxiety disorder	13.4 (8.06–21.4)
Obsessive–compulsive disorder	30.4 (16.3–49.4)
Panic disorder	3.73 (0.87–14.7)
Mixed anxiety and depression	9.54 (5.84–15.2)
Post-traumatic stress disorder	7.79 (3.60–16.1)
Attention deficit hyperactivity disorder	6.88 (13.2–29.0)
Eating disorder	17.0 (6.23–38.7)
Probable psychosis	28.5 (8.56–63.0)
Currently taking a psychoactive medication[b]	12.4 (7.88–19.0)

[a]Weighted to account for survey design.
[b]Small numbers make it difficult to assess HSI according to individual drug use with any precision.
APMS, Adult Psychiatric Morbidity Survey; CIS-R, revised Clinical Interview Schedule; CI, confidence interval; HSI, Heaviness of Smoking Index.

the GHQ-12 the proportion was 7%, in those currently taking a psychoactive medication 14%, and in those who also reported a longstanding mental health condition 17% (Fig 2.3). Similar observations apply in APMS data (Table 2.6), which show a particularly high prevalence of heavy addiction among those with obsessive–compulsive disorder and probable psychosis.

2.7 Association between cigarette consumption and mental disorders

We examined whether HSE and APMS data support previous reports of an association between dependence on tobacco and severity of mental disorder.[1,3] Table 2.7 shows the proportion of HSE and APMS participants grouped by smoking status and daily cigarette consumption who meet the case definition criteria for the available measures of mental disorder. As can be seen, smokers are much more likely to have a mental disorder than never smokers and, in most cases, ex-smokers. In general, the greater the number of cigarettes smoked per day, the higher the prevalence of mental disorder in that group.

Figure 2.4 shows smoking status and daily cigarette consumption in APMS participants grouped by CIS-R score, and also demonstrates a clear dose–response relationship between the severity of mental disorder (indicated by CIS-R score) and smoking behaviour. The higher the CIS-R score the greater the proportion of participants who are smokers, and the higher the average daily cigarette consumption.

2.8 Proportion of cigarettes smoked by people with a mental disorder

Previous analysis of APMS data suggested that 42% of all cigarettes consumed in England are smoked by people with a mental disorder.[9] However, this analysis used an inclusive definition of mental disorder, and included people with a dependence on alcohol or illicit drugs, those with problem gambling and those who had made a suicide attempt in the past year. Using the less inclusive definition of mental disorder used throughout this report, 33% of all cigarettes are smoked by people with a mental disorder. The majority of these, 29% of all cigarettes, are smoked by people with a common mental disorder who scored 12+ on the CIS-R.

2.9 Quitting behaviour

Although people with mental disorders are more likely to be smokers and more likely to be heavily addicted to cigarettes than those without, data from the HSE

Table 2.7 Proportion of participants with mental disorders by smoking status (HSE and APMS data)

Indicator of mental disorder	Never smokers	Ex-smokers	0–10 cigs/day	11–20 cigs/day	21+ cigs/day
GHQ-12 score 3+ (HSE)	16.9 (15.6–18.3)	18.8 (17.1–20.7)	25.6 (22.2–29.4)	26.6 (22.9–30.7)	29.2 (22.2–37.5)
CIS-R 12+ (APMS)	12.8 (11.5–14.3)	12.6 (11.4–14.0)	22.3 (19.0–25.9)	21.0 (17.9–24.6)	33.1 (26.1–40.9)
Longstanding mental disorder (HSE)	3.28 (2.66–4.06)	3.09 (2.37–4.01)	4.88 (3.50–6.77)	8.65 (6.64–11.2)	17.3 (11.9–24.3)
Any mental disorder (APMS)	15.5 (14.0–17.1)	15.3 (13.8–16.6)	25.0 (21.5–28.9)	24.7 (21.5–28.4)	37.1 (29.8–44.9)
Taken a psychoactive medication in last 7 days (HSE)	4.10 (3.51–4.79)	6.18 (5.22–7.30)	5.04 (3.76–6.71)	7.96 (6.11–10.3)	12.8 (8.41–18.9)
Currently taking a psychoactive medication (APMS)	4.86 (4.04–5.85)	4.71 (4.07–5.44)	6.71 (5.12–8.76)	9.40 (7.25–12.1)	13.5 (9.19–19.3)

APMS, Adult Psychiatric Morbidity Survey; CIS-R, revised Clinical Interview Schedule; GHQ-12, 12-item General Health Questionnaire; HSE, Health Survey for England.

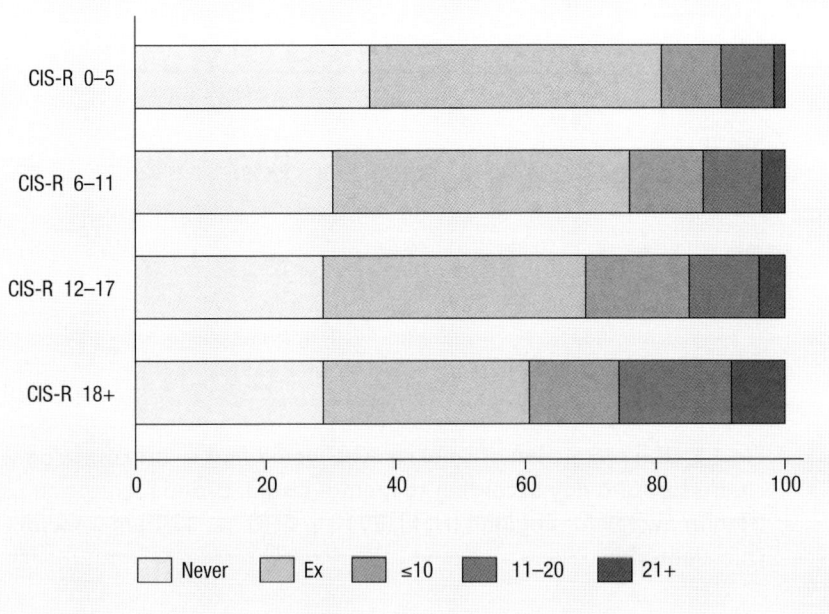

Fig 2.4 Smoking status and daily cigarette consumption by increasing severity of mental illness (Adult Psychiatric Morbidity Surveys (APMS), 2007[5]). CIS-R, revised Clinical Interview Schedule.

indicate that they are no less likely to want to quit smoking. When asked whether they would like to give up smoking altogether, 66% of all smokers in the HSE responded positively, as did 69% of smokers taking a psychoactive medication, 71% of smokers scoring 3 or more on the GHQ-12 and 61% of smokers reporting a longstanding mental health condition.

However, smokers with mental disorders were more likely to report that they expected to find quitting difficult, and were less likely to expect to succeed, than smokers without these disorders. When asked how easy or difficult they would find it to go without cigarettes for a whole day, 55% of all smokers completing the HSE reported that they would find it fairly or very difficult. A significantly higher proportion, 79%, of smokers reporting a longstanding mental health condition believed that they would find such abstinence fairly or very difficult, as did 72% of smokers taking a psychoactive medication. Of smokers scoring 3 or more on the GHQ-12, 62% reported that they would find quitting for a day difficult, although this proportion was not significantly different from that in all smokers (Fig 2.5).

This expectation of greater difficulty quitting smoking is consistent with the observation of lower quit ratios in those with mental disorders in the HSE. Among all HSE participants, approximately 56% of ever-smokers had quit smoking by the time of the survey. However, although the quit ratio among

Smoking and mental health

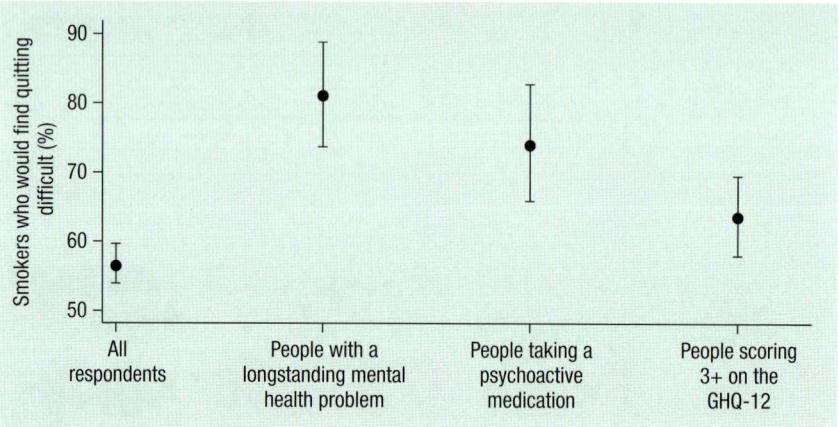

Fig 2.5 The proportion of smokers who would find it difficult to go without cigarettes for a day according to mental disorders and medication use (Health Survey for England (HSE), 2010[4]). GHQ-12, 12-item General Health Questionnaire.

Table 2.8 Quit ratios according to psychiatric diagnosis and medication use (HSE, 2010[4])

	Percentage current smokers (95% CI)	Percentage ex-smokers (95% CI)	Quit ratio (95% CI)
All participants	20.1 (18.9–21.3)	25.2 (24.1–26.4)	0.56 (0.54–0.57)
Participants reporting a longstanding mental health condition	37.4 (31.9–43.1)	19.0 (15.0–23.7)	0.34 (0.27–0.40)
Participants scoring 3+ on the GHQ-12	27.3 (24.7–30.0)	25.1 (22.8–27.6)	0.48 (0.44–0.51)
Participants currently taking a psychoactive medication	26.9 (22.8–31.3)	31.3 (27.3–35.5)	0.53 (0.47–0.58)

CI, confidence interval; GHQ-12, 12-item General Health Questionnaire; HSE, Health Survey for England.

people using psychoactive medications was similar at 53%, the ratio in those with GHQ-12 scores of 3 or more was significantly lower at 48% and in those with a mental disorder also significantly lower at 34% (Table 2.8).

2.10 Delivery of smoking cessation interventions

Brief smoking cessation advice delivered during routine general practice consultations has been shown to be effective in increasing cessation rates in the general population,[27] and is one of the most cost-effective means to reduce the burden of smoking.[28] Similarly, the use of NRT,[29] bupropion[30] or varenicline[31] significantly increases the chances of a quit attempt succeeding.

THIN data demonstrate that, after taking into account differences in age, sex, socioeconomic status and a history of smoking-related chronic disease, smokers with some mental disorders are generally (and in most categories, significantly) more likely than the general population of smokers to have had delivery of advice to quit smoking during the past year recorded in their medical notes[32] (Fig 2.6). Similar findings applied to prescribing of smoking cessation medications, which was also significantly more likely to occur in most mental disorder diagnostic and medication use groups than in smokers without mental disorders (Fig 2.7).

Although these differences probably reflect in large part the effect of the recently-introduced QOF incentive for GPs to offer smoking cessation advice and support to smokers with certain mental disorders and the eligibility of many patients with mental disorders for free prescriptions, these findings indicate

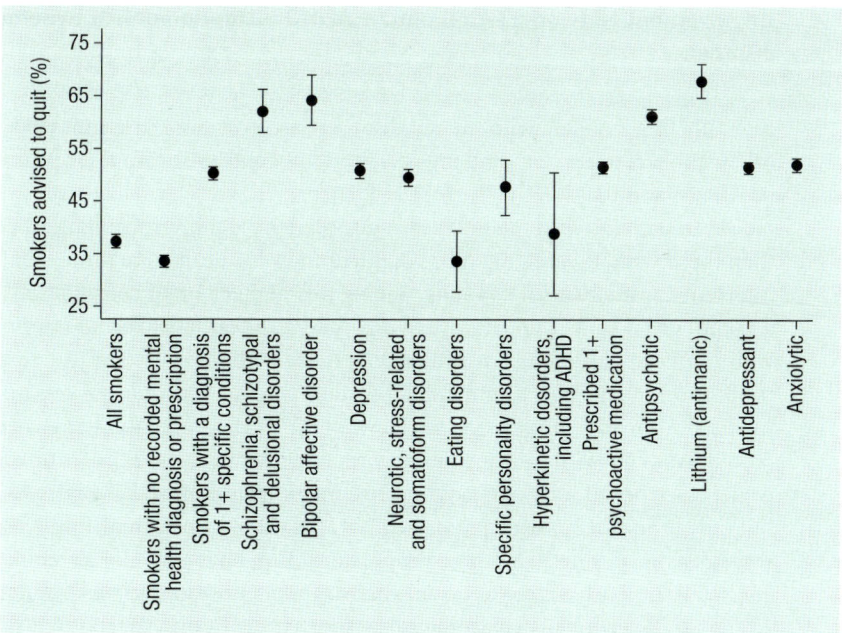

Fig 2.6 The proportion of smokers advised to quit according to mental disorders and medication use (The Health Improvement Network (THIN) data[6]). ADHD, attention deficit hyperactivity disorder.

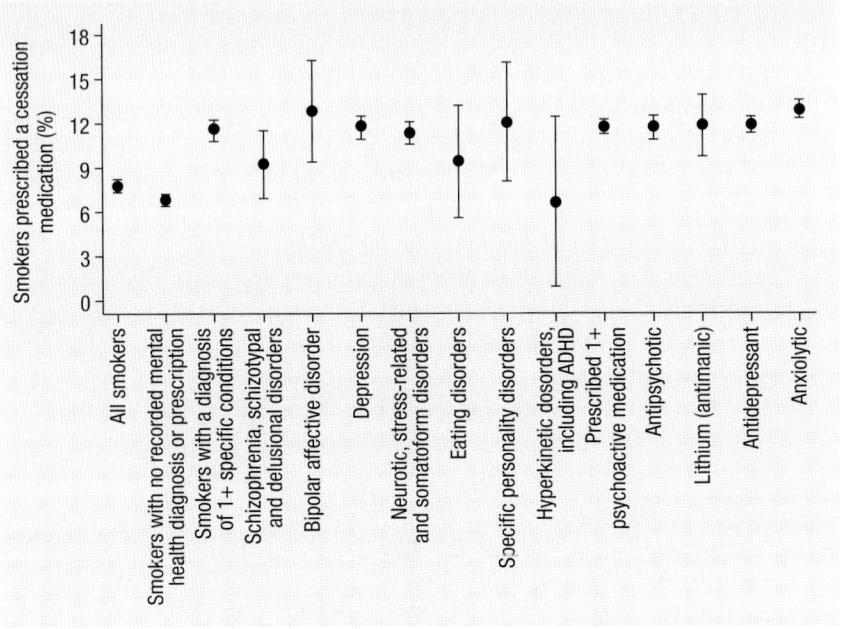

Fig 2.7 The proportion of smokers prescribed a smoking cessation medication according to mental disorder and medication use (The Health Improvement Network (THIN) data[6]). ADHD, attention deficit hyperactivity disorder.

generally that smokers with mental disorders are now over 80% more likely than other smokers to receive smoking cessation interventions from their primary care providers, and that NRT is the most widely prescribed pharmacotherapy. However, patients with mental health disorders have more consultations per year than those without, creating more opportunities for healthcare professionals to intervene on the issue of smoking. Taking this higher rate of consultations into account, given equal opportunity to do so, GPs appear less likely to intervene with smokers with mental disorders than those without.[32] Overall, the total proportion of smokers with mental disorders who are prescribed a cessation medication in any one year remains low; in the THIN population approximately 50% of smokers with one or more recorded mental health diagnoses or who had been prescribed at least one psychoactive medication were given advice to quit, but only around 12% were prescribed NRT, bupropion or varenicline. Although some discrepancy between these proportions is inevitable, as not all smokers advised to quit are willing to do so whereas others prepared to make a quit attempt will decline pharmacological support, these figures suggest that there is a large opportunity for improvement in the number of smokers with mental disorders who are offered and take up evidence-based cessation interventions in primary care.

2.11 Supplementary APMS survey data on special populations

In the 1996 APMS supplementary survey of those living in institutions catering for people with mental illness three categories of mental disorder were examined: those with a diagnosis of schizophrenia, delusional or schizoaffective disorders (around 70% of the sample); affective psychoses (mania and bipolar affective disorder – around 8%); and 'neurotic disorders' (those with a diagnosis of generalised anxiety disorder, depressive episode, mixed anxiety and depressive disorder, phobia, obsessive–compulsive disorder and panic disorder – around 8%). Of the remainder, 5% had other mental disorders and in 9% data were insufficient to enable classification. Smoking prevalence among those with these disorders is shown in Table 2.9, and reflects rates approximately three times higher than the 27% in the general population at the time.[23] Among homeless people, smoking prevalence was also high at 71% overall, and 84% among residents of night shelters (84%) and 91% in those sleeping rough. Among prisoners surveyed in 1997, 82% reported smoking, when the prevalence of smoking in the general population was still 27%.

Table 2.9 Prevalence of smoking in special population groups

Sample and diagnosis	Year of survey	N[a]	Smoking prevalence (95% CI)[b]
Institutional sample			
Schizophrenia, delusional and schizoaffective disorders	1994	856	81.8 (77.5–85.3)
Affective psychosis	1994	101	78.2 (64.1–87.9)
Neurotic disorders	1994	78	73.9 (60.4–84.2)
Homeless people	1994	1,166	71.2 (67.6–74.8)
Prisoners	1997	3,107	81.8 (80.4–83.1)

[a]Unweighted (previous published data from the institutional survey have been based on a smaller subset of participants who also provided information on alcohol and drug use).
[b]Weighted to account for survey design.
CI, confidence interval.

2.12 Summary

> - Smoking is around twice as common among people with mental disorders, and more so in those with more severe disease.
> - Up to 3 million smokers in the UK, 30% of all smokers, have evidence of mental disorder and up to 1 million with longstanding disease.

> A third of all cigarettes smoked in England are smoked by people with a mental disorder.
> In contrast to the marked decline in smoking prevalence in the general population, smoking among those with mental disorder has changed little, if at all, over the past 20 years.
> Smokers with mental disorders are just as likely to want to quit as those without, but are more likely to be heavily addicted to smoking and to anticipate difficulty quitting smoking, and are historically much less likely to succeed in any quit attempt.
> Over the course of a year, smokers with mental disorders are more likely to receive advice from their GP to quit smoking, and be prescribed cessation medications, but this reflects the increased frequency of their consultations. Overall, only a minority receive cessation pharmacotherapy.

References

1 Meltzer H, Gill B, Hinds K, Petticrew M. *OPCS Surveys of Psychiatric Morbidity in Great Britain, Report 6: Economic activity and social functioning of residents with psychiatric disorders.* London: HMSO, 1996.

2 Lasser K, Boyd JW, Woolhandler S, et al. Smoking and mental illness. *Journal of the American Medical Association* 2000;284:2606–10.

3 Farrell M, Howes S, Taylor C, et al. Substance misuse and psychiatric comorbidity: An overview of the opcs national psychiatric morbidity survey. *Addictive Behaviors* 1998;23:909–18.

4 The NHS Information Centre. *Health Survey for England.* www.ic.nhs.uk/statistics-and-data-collections/health-and-lifestyles-related-surveys/health-survey-for-england [Accessed 12 November 2012]

5 The NHS Information Centre. *Adult Psychiatric Morbidity in England, 2007: results of a household survey.* www.ic.nhs.uk/pubs/psychiatricmorbidity07 [Accessed 12 November 2012]

6 Epidemiology and Pharmacology Information Core. THIN data. http://csdmruk.cegedim.com/our-data/statistics.shtml [Accessed 12 November 2012}

7 Goldberg D. *Manual of the General Health Questionnaire.* Windsor: NFER Publishing, 1978.

8 Heatherton T, Kozlowski L, Frecker R, Rickert W, Robinson J. Measuring the heaviness of smoking: using self-reported time to the first cigarette of the day and number of cigarettes smoked per day. *British Journal of Addiction* 1989;84:791–9.

9 McManus S, Meltzer H, Campion J. *Cigarette smoking and mental health in England: Data from the Adult Psychiatric Morbidity Survey 2007.* London: National Centre for Social Research, 2010.

10 Lewis G, Pelosi A, Araya R, Dunn G. Measuring psychiatric disorder in the community; a standardised assessment for use by lay interviewers. *Psychological Medicine* 1992;22:465–86.

11 Brewin C, Rose S, Andrews B, et al. Brief screening instrument for post-traumatic stress disorder. *British Journal of Psychiatry* 2002;181:158–62.

12 World Health Organization. *Adult ADHD Self-Report Scale-V1.1 (ASRS-V1.1) Screen. WHO Composite International Diagnostic Interview.* Geneva: WHO, 2003.

13 Morgan JF RF, Lacey JH. The SCOFF questionnaire: assessment of a new screening tool for eating disorders. *British Medical Journal* 1999;319:1467–8.

14 Economic and Social Data Service. OPCS Surveys of Psychiatric Morbidity: Institutions Sample, 1994. www.esds.ac.uk/findingData/snDescription.asp?sn=3585 [Accessed 15 November 2012]

15 Economic and Social Data Service. OPCS Survey of Psychiatric Morbidity among Homeless People, 1994. www.esds.ac.uk/findingData/snDescription.asp?sn=3642 [Accessed 15 November 2012]

16 Economic and Social Data Service. ONS Survey of Psychiatric Morbidity among Prisoners in England and Wales, 1997. www.esds.ac.uk/findingData/snDescription.asp?sn=4320 [Accessed 15 November 2012]

17 INPS. http://www.inps4.co.uk [Accessed 25 January 2012]

18 Szatkowski L, Lewis S, McNeill A, Huang Y, Coleman T. Can data from primary care medical records be used to monitor national smoking prevalence? *Journal of Epidemiology and Community Health* 2012;66:791–5.

19 NHS Connecting for Health. Read Codes. www.connectingforhealth.nhs.uk/systemsandservices/data/readcodes [Accessed 12 November 2012]

20 *British National Formulary* No. 63 (March 2012). http://bnf.org/bnf/index.htm [Accessed 5 August 2012]

21 Szatkowski L, McNeill A, Lewis S, Coleman T. A comparison of patient recall of smoking cessation advice with advice recorded in electronic medical records. *BMC Public Health* 2011;11:291.

22 Langley T, Szatkowski L, Gibson J, *et al*. Validation of The Health Improvement Network (THIN) primary care database for monitoring prescriptions for smoking cessation medications *Pharmacoepidemiology and Drug Safety* 2010;19:586–90.

23 Dunstan S. *General Lifestyle Survey Overview: A report on the 2010 General Lifestyle Survey*. Newport: Office for National Statistics, 2012.

24 Office for National Statistics. Population Estimates for UK, England and Wales, Scotland and Northern Ireland – mid 2010. www.ons.gov.uk/ons/publications/re-reference-tables.html?edition=tcm%3A77–231847 [Accessed 12 November 2012]

25 Action on Smoking and Health. *Smoking Statistics: Who Smokes and How Much*. London: Action on Smoking and Health, 2007.

26 Communities and Local Government. Indices of Deprivation 2007. http://webarchive.nationalarchives.gov.uk/20100410180038/http://communities.gov.uk/communities/neighbourhoodrenewal/deprivation/deprivation07 [Accessed 25 January 2012]

27 Stead LF, Bergson G, Lancaster T. Physician advice for smoking cessation. *Cochrane Database of Systematic Reviews* 2008;(2):CD000165.

28 Flack S, Taylor M, Trueman P. *Cost-Effectiveness of Interventions for Smoking Cessation*. York: York Health Economics Consortium, 2007.

29 Stead LF, Perera R, Bullen C, Mant D, Lancaster T. Nicotine replacement therapy for smoking cessation. *Cochrane Database of Systematic Reviews* 2008;(1):CD000146.

30 Hughes JR, Stead LF, Lancaster T. Antidepressants for smoking cessation. *Cochrane Database of Systematic Reviews* 2007;(1):CD000031.

31 Cahill K, Stead LF, Lancaster T. Nicotine receptor partial agonists for smoking cessation. *Cochrane Database of Systematic Reviews* 2008;(3):CD006103.

32 Szatkowski L, McNeill A. The delivery of smoking cessation interventions to primary care patients with mental health problems. *Addiction* In press.

3 Neurobiological and behavioural mechanisms linking smoking and mental disorders

Although the prevalence of smoking among people with mental disorders is high, and as outlined in Chapter 2 has proved relatively refractory to change, the mechanisms underlying this association, and in particular the direction of causation between smoking and mental illness, remain poorly understood. This chapter reviews some of the biological mechanisms that may be responsible for the association between smoking and mental disorders.

3.1 Mechanisms of nicotine addiction

There is widespread agreement that nicotine is the principal addictive component of tobacco smoke. Behavioural studies with experimental animals have provided convincing evidence that nicotine has the behavioural properties of drugs of dependence, because nicotine serves as a reinforcer in self-administration studies,[1,2] and abrupt withdrawal after a period of continuous infusion evokes a withdrawal syndrome, which is reversed by the re-administration of nicotine.[3,4] The behavioural changes evoked by nicotine withdrawal in this paradigm are thought to model important components of the abstinence syndrome experienced by many smokers when they first quit smoking.[5,6] Neurobiological studies have also shown that nicotine acts on neural pathways within the brain that have been implicated in reward and reinforcement. In experimental animals, injections of nicotine delivered non-contingently (ie by an experimenter) or contingently (by self-administration) stimulate the release of dopamine in both the shell and core subdivisions of the nucleus accumbens.[7–9] Repeated daily administration of the drug results in sensitisation of its effects on dopamine (DA) overflow in the core subdivision of the accumbens.[10–12] This effect is independent of contingency. However, repeated self-administration of nicotine across days also results in sensitisation of its effect on DA overflow in the shell subdivision of the accumbens.[9] Sensitisation of these pathways is a property of drugs of dependence of different pharmacological groups, and has been implicated in the transition from simple reinforcement to the compulsive drug-seeking and drug-taking behaviour that characterises dependence.[13,14]

Although it is clear that nicotine has the neurobiological and behavioural properties of a drug of dependence, when compared with many drugs of dependence used illicitly its reinforcing properties are weak and appear insufficient to account for the powerful dependence on tobacco experienced by most habitual smokers.[15] Furthermore, the therapeutic nicotine preparations commonly used to aid cessation are neither strongly effective in this regard nor commonly subject to abuse. These observations have led to the conclusion that the tobacco smoke vehicle, through which most people dose themselves with nicotine, may also play an important part in addiction to tobacco smoking.

There are a number of components of tobacco smoke that could enhance the addictive properties of nicotine. Some of these inhibit the enzyme monoamine oxidase, which metabolises dopamine in the brain, thereby enhancing the rewarding effects evoked by release of this monoamine.[16–18] Studies in experimental animals have confirmed that inhibition of monoamine oxidase potentiates nicotine self-administration.[19–21] Other studies have focused on the role of non-pharmacological factors such as environmental or conditioned stimuli associated with the delivery of nicotine, both of which significantly enhance self-administration of nicotine.[22–24] Sensorimotor stimuli also seem to be important factors in the development of tobacco dependence,[25] particularly among highly dependent smokers.[26] These observations have led Rose[27] to suggest that non-nicotinic factors play a pivotal role in tobacco dependence. Similarly, these and other results have led Caggiula and colleagues[28] to propose a dual reinforcement model of tobacco dependence that relies on both the primary reinforcing properties of nicotine itself, and enhancement by nicotine of the reinforcing salience of other sensory or contextual stimuli, paired with the delivery of the drug.

3.2 Models of association and sources of evidence

One possible mechanism of association between smoking and mental disorders is the self-medication model, whereby smoking is used to alleviate symptoms, particularly those of negative affect and impaired cognition,[29,30] eg individuals with negative affect may turn to substance use, including tobacco, to alleviate emotional distress,[29] whereas individuals with attentional and learning deficits may use tobacco to help them overcome these limitations. Cultural and social beliefs, eg a belief that smoking is an effective anxiolytic or antidepressant, even in the absence of a true effect, may also contribute to this process. Alternatively, smoking could be a causal risk factor for the development of mental illness, although it is also possible that the association is due to confounding by other factors, eg genetic traits, that independently influence both smoking and mental illness. In addition it is possible that the nature of the association changes with chronicity of exposure.

3.2.1 Genetic evidence

Twin studies have long been used to explore the genetic and environmental influences underlying human phenotypes such as smoking, because they provide an opportunity to separate the contributions of several latent sources of variance: genetic factors, environmental factors shared by both twins and environmental factors that are unique to one twin. This is accomplished by comparing the phenotypic correlation of monozygotic twins, who share all their genes, to that of dizygotic twins, who share on average half of their segregating genes identical by descent. If monozygotic twins are more similar to one another than dizygotic twins, genetic influences are likely to be an important contributor to variation in that phenotype. A straightforward bivariate extension of the standard twin model enables researchers to investigate whether smoking is genetically and/or environmentally correlated with other disorders. This method can be used to quantify shared latent genetic factors, and can be followed up by molecular genetic studies aimed at identifying specific genes or variants that underlie the latent factor. Genetic evidence specific to associations between nicotine use and selected mental disorders is summarised in later sections.

3.2.2 Animal models

Much of the evidence from studies in animals derives from studies testing the hypothesis that nicotine exerts effects in the brain which ameliorate the symptoms of underlying mental disorders, and thus provide a form of self-medication.[30,31] Nicotine deprivation produces withdrawal effects that often include impairments in mood and cognition,[32,33] but nicotine may also have beneficial effects on mood and cognition that are independent of its ability to reverse nicotine withdrawal symptoms,[34] eg nicotinic acetylcholine receptors (nAChRs) have been implicated in the pathophysiology of depression[35] and nicotine and nAChR agonists have demonstrated antidepressant effects in animal models of the disease.[36,37] In addition, nicotine stimulates dopamine release in the mesolimbic system, and chronic nicotine administration may sensitise this effect (ie lower the threshold of stimulation needed for release), particularly in stressful situations.[38] Reduced bioavailability of dopamine in this region of the brain has been implicated in causing the anhedonia associated with depressive disorders.[39] In addition, the effects of nicotine on the hypothalamic–pituitary–adrenal (HPA) axis appear to play an important role in the anxiolytic effects of nicotine in response to acute and chronic stress.[32]

Cholinergic innervation of areas of the brain involved in the stress response, most notably the HPA axis, is probably critical in modulating anxiety and there are a large variety of nAChR subtypes expressed in these pathways. Animal studies have also demonstrated that nicotine stimulates the release of allopregnanolone and neuropeptide Y, both of which act to reduce anxiety.[40,41]

Finally, studies have demonstrated that attentional processes and other cognitive functions (eg concentration) are mediated by cholinergic systems in the prefrontal, occipital and parietal cortices of the brain, as well as the amygdala, hippocampus and anterior cingulate cortex.[42] The nAChRs are widely expressed in these areas of the brain[43] and experimental manipulation of these receptors affects attention-related task performance in animal studies.[44] Several studies have indicated that nAChRs, and specifically the α_7 subtype in the hippocampus, may be crucial in sensory gating.[45] Deficits in sensory gating are characteristic in people with schizophrenia and studies have shown that nicotine enhances sensory gating processes in people with this disorder.[46]

3.2.3 Social and psychosocial mechanisms

Psychosocial risk factors for tobacco use among smokers with a mental disorder are important and often neglected relative to biological factors. Theories of psychosocial risk for tobacco use typically group variables into four conceptual domains according to whether they are intrapersonal (eg mood related), interpersonal (both family and peer related), behavioural (eg rebelliousness, impulsiveness) or organisational (eg cultural factors, organisational norms and practices). Of note, there are many known psychosocial risk factors for tobacco addiction in the general population that are also associated with mental illness, such as low income, limited education, unemployment, manual and unskilled occupations, and being single or divorced. These general psychosocial risk factors complicate the isolation of those who might be susceptible to mental disorders. In addition, there is a wide range of mental disorders of varying severity, medication and co-morbidity, and therefore there are many subtypes within the broad category of mental disorders.

Prospective studies of adolescents and young adults in the general population have identified several psychosocial risk factors associated with initiation of tobacco use and escalation to regular smoking, including higher perceived benefits of tobacco use relative to risks, low levels of parental support and monitoring, parental use of tobacco, social networks of tobacco-using peers, and poor school performance.[47,48] However, very few of these risk factors have been examined in studies of the association between tobacco use and mental illness.

3.3 Depression and anxiety

The association between tobacco use and depression, and to a lesser extent the association with anxiety, is widely recognised. Evidence is available on these associations from a range of sources.

3.3.1 Evidence from genetic studies

A study of a population-based sample of female twins born in Virginia, USA, which used a co-twin control design and bivariate twin model,[49] found that the best-fitting model indicated that lifetime smoking and major depression were substantially genetically correlated. No environmental correlation between smoking and depression was detected. Similarly, Korhonen and colleagues,[50] in a sample of Finnish twins, reported a moderate genetic correlation and a more modest non-shared environmental correlation that was not statistically significant.

Interestingly, the genetic relationship between depression and tobacco dependence is often found to appear stronger than the relationship between depression and smoking, eg Lyons and colleagues[51] reported a modest genetic correlation between depression and regular tobacco use, but a strong correlation between depression and tobacco dependence in men. Another study also reported modest genetic correlations between regular tobacco use and depression but slightly higher correlations between depression and tobacco dependence.[52] Modest environmental correlations were detected for both smoking-related phenotypes.[52] Such studies suggest that, although liability to smoking initiation is largely independent of liability to depression – perhaps more a function of peer influences or externalising tendencies – once smoking has been initiated, an individual's degree of dependence is related to his or her genetic liability to depression. Consequently, individuals with a history (or family history) of depression could establish higher levels of dependence, and might find smoking cessation more difficult than others.

Although results vary between studies, most findings support the existence of modest-to-moderate genetic correlations between major depression (or depressive symptoms) and smoking and/or tobacco dependence. Molecular genetic studies can be designed to identify the genes within which variation contributes to liability to both phenotypes. Such genes might be related to personality constructs (eg locus of control, neuroticism), or to neural systems such as dopaminergic or glutamatergic neurotransmission, which are both involved in depression and the establishment or maintenance of tobacco dependence.[53]

3.3.2 Evidence from animal studies

Evidence that nicotine has antidepressant-like effects is available from a range of animal models including the forced swim test,[54,56] and in studies of rats with an inbred[57,58] or induced behavioural phenotype characteristic of depression.[59] Nicotine also attenuates the reduction in sucrose preference evoked by chronic exposure to an unpredictable mild stressor,[60] which is thought to reflect the development of anhedonia (a reduced ability to respond to a pleasurable reward), a major symptom of depression. This evidence suggests that nicotine has antidepressant-like activity in experimental animal models, and that it may act preferentially in animals which are particularly susceptible to a depression-like behavioural phenotype.[59]

Nicotine injections also enhance the ability of the brain to respond to pleasurable stimuli or events, and this reward enhancement has been observed following both experimenter-administered[61] and self-administered[62,63] nicotine. In intracranial self-stimulation, a procedure in which animals are trained to perform a task that results in stimulation of small electrodes located in pathways within the brain that mediate reward, nicotine injections decrease the electrical current required to maintain responding,[64,65] whereas abrupt withdrawal of nicotine, after a period of chronic infusion, increases the current required.[3,5] The withdrawal-evoked increase in brain reward sensitivity induced by nicotine self-administration persists for many days.[66] These findings indicate that the antidepressant properties of nicotine may arise from its ability to enhance mood by altering the way in which it is influenced by positive and negative stimuli, and that nicotine withdrawal may exacerbate the influence of negative stimuli. If the administration of the drug is controlled by the individual, its reward-enhancing properties may be increased and prolonged and may, therefore, contribute significantly to the addictive properties of the drug.

There is evidence that mesolimbic dopaminergic neurons play a pivotal role in tobacco dependence (see Balfour[15] for a review), and that anhedonia and depression are associated with reduced mesolimbic DA release.[67] Similar mechanisms are thought to contribute to the psychopathology of nicotine withdrawal.[68] Thus, it seems likely that increases in DA release evoked in the nucleus accumbens, the principal terminal field of the mesolimbic dopaminergic system, not only mediate the reinforcing properties of nicotine in general but also contribute specifically to the amelioration of anhedonia in depression. This hypothesis provides an explanation for the role of depression in tobacco dependence that has clear face validity. However, it hides a conundrum. Many depressed patients smoke heavily, in a way that is likely to generate blood nicotine levels which desensitise many of the neuronal nicotinic receptors in the brain and in turn mediate the effects of nicotine on DA release.[15,69] Thus, the hypothesis above does not provide a complete explanation for the mechanism through which tobacco smoke may serve as an antidepressant.

In some of the forced swim test studies[56,58] nicotine was given either acutely or repeatedly as a subcutaneous injection, a route of administration that is likely to result in stimulation of neuronal nicotinic receptors. In other studies nicotine was given in drinking water[57] or by continuous subcutaneous infusion,[70] thus maintaining blood nicotine concentrations at a level that desensitises nicotinic receptors but, perhaps, models more closely the pattern of exposure experienced by heavy smokers. Interestingly, there is evidence that nicotinic receptor antagonists also demonstrate antidepressant-like activity in this test,[54] which supports the conclusion that desensitisation of neuronal nicotinic receptors may also exert a beneficial effect on mood in depressed patients.

Compounds such as cytisine and varenicline, which are partial agonists at the neuronal $\alpha_4\beta_2$ nicotinic receptor subtype that is most closely implicated in tobacco dependence, are also reported to exhibit antidepressant-like activity in a number of rodent models.[70,71] These findings provide further support for the hypothesis that compounds that desensitise neuronal nicotinic receptors have putative efficacy as antidepressants. They also imply that this component of their pharmacological activity may be important to their efficacy as aids for smoking cessation, especially in smokers in whom depression contributes significantly to the addiction itself or the severity of the abstinence syndrome.

Exposure to a stressful stimulus is commonly an intrinsic component of rodent models of depression. Furthermore, generalised anxiety disorder is a common co-morbidity in patients who experience depression.[72] The results of some animal studies suggest that nicotine has anxiolytic-like activity in a number of models[73–75] although this is not a consistent finding.[69,76] Other studies have reported that nicotine also has anxiogenic properties in the elevated plus-maze test.[77,78] Caldarone et al[77] showed that this anxiogenic response was more marked in female mice and suggested that this observation may provide a model for the increased vulnerability to relapse evoked by exposure to stressful or depressogenic stimuli. Other studies in rats suggest that the anxiolytic response to nicotine is observed only after repeated administration of the drug, and that acute nicotine is anxiogenic.[79] This last observation is consistent with evidence that acute nicotine stimulates corticosterone release in rats but that this response develops tolerance when daily injections of nicotine are given for periods exceeding 5 days.[80]

Other studies support the conclusion that exposure to a stressful stimulus evokes nicotine-seeking behaviour because, in self-administration studies with rats or mice, exposure to a stimulus of this nature reinstates responding in animals in which the response has been extinguished.[81,82] Thus, the data taken together suggest that stress may play a significant role in strengthening the reinforcing properties of nicotine, and this may be related to an anxiolytic-like property of the drug. By contrast, nicotine withdrawal is reported to potentiate the effects of stress in at least one model.[83] Thus, it seems reasonable to propose that exposure to a stressful stimulus or the presence of an underlying stress-related psychopathology may exacerbate the adverse effects of tobacco withdrawal and enhance relapse.[84]

3.3.3 Evidence from human studies

Several studies have investigated the effect of nicotine administration on mood.[85,86] Kalman[85] found little consistent evidence for a beneficial effect of nicotine on mood that was independent of an effect due to the reversal of withdrawal symptoms, and a subsequent meta-analysis confirmed this conclusion.[86] However, interesting interactions between nicotine and other variables on mood including psychiatric diagnosis and subclinical affective syndromes have been reported. In a series of small laboratory studies that included people with major depression, Salin-Pascual and colleagues[87–89] found that a moderate-strength nicotine patch applied for several days improved mood relative to placebo patch in both depressed and non-depressed non-smokers. As non-smokers were tested, the effect cannot be attributed to reversal of the nicotine withdrawal syndrome. In a more recent investigation with non-smokers with major depression, Cox and colleagues[90] found improvements in mood among participants in both the nicotine and placebo patch condition. McClernon and colleagues[91] found that a nicotine patch worn for 4 weeks by subclinically depressed non-smoking participants improved mood over the first 3 weeks of the trial, whereas participants assigned to the placebo patch condition did not report any improvements in mood.[92]

In a study of non-smoking adults with attention deficit hyperactivity disorder (ADHD), nicotine (but not placebo) decreased depression scores after 15 days of administration.[93] In a field study using real-time data collection, Jamner and colleagues[94] found that both smokers and non-smokers high in trait hostility (assessed at baseline) reported lower levels of angry mood and greater wellbeing when wearing a nicotine patch but not when wearing a placebo patch. Non-smokers reported that angry mood was experienced for 23% of a day in which they wore a placebo patch, compared with 14% when using a nicotine patch; for smokers the proportions were 55% and 32% respectively. In a laboratory study, Kassel and Unrod[95] found support for their hypothesis that smoking has a calming or stress-relieving effect only (or especially) among highly anxious smokers and only in combination with a stimulus that distracts them from the source of stress. Taken together, although limited in number, these studies suggest that the mood effects of nicotine may be more apparent in psychiatrically impaired subgroups of smokers, including under stressful and other conditions.

Studies of negative affect as a risk factor for tobacco use have also investigated additional risk factors. Adolescents with negative affect or anxiety are more likely to associate with peers who smoke,[96–99] which in turn predicts smoking initiation and progression to regular use.[100] Adolescents with higher levels of depression may also be more sensitive to peer behaviour, more likely to select non-conventional peers or both.[96] Parental attachment problems (including poor communication and trust between parents and offspring) and adverse childhood events (such as socioeconomic disadvantage or physical abuse), as reported by adolescents, are also associated with increased risks of both depressive symptoms and tobacco use.[97]

Prospective studies of the temporal association between depressive affect and both smoking initiation and progression to regular tobacco use indicate that depressive affect precedes smoking initiation, although the evidence is somewhat mixed, and the relationship may be bidirectional,[101] eg Audrain-McGovern and colleagues[96] found that higher depression and anxiety scores increased risk of smoking initiation, and that higher depression symptom levels were associated with earlier smoking initiation, whereas no relationship was reported by Wang and colleagues.[102] In a study using real-time data collection, Whalen and colleagues found that negative affect preceded daily occurrences of smoking.[103] Among young adult smokers, Breslau and colleagues[104] found that a history of major depression predicted progression to dependence and more severe levels of dependence; however, a history of anxiety disorder did not predict progression. These investigators also found that a history of tobacco dependence predicted onset of major depression. McKenzie and colleagues[105] found that higher depression and anxiety symptoms predicted progression to tobacco dependence in young adulthood,[102,106] whereas Audrain-McGovern *et al*[96] found that regular smoking was associated with a decrease in depression symptoms, consistent with a self-medication model. Further evidence on these associations is provided in Chapter 4. Individuals with major depression have been found to have increased vulnerability to a mood disorder relapse during abstinence from smoking, particularly those with histories of recurrent depression.[107] However, history of depression does not appear to influence the likelihood of successful smoking cessation.[108]

3.4 Schizophrenia

The prevalence of tobacco smoking among patients with schizophrenia is extremely high (see Chapter 2), as are levels of dependence on tobacco in this patient group.[46]

3.4.1 Evidence from genetic studies

The relationship between smoking and schizophrenia has rarely been explored in a genetic epidemiological framework. Thus, it remains unclear whether a common genetic and/or environmental liability contributes to the association. One study of twins discordant for schizophrenia found that unaffected co-twins were more likely to smoke, more likely to experience some withdrawal symptoms and less successful at quitting compared with control individuals.[109] The authors concluded that familial factors – encompassing both genetic and environmental factors – contributed to the phenotypic association between smoking and schizophrenia. Molecular genetic studies suggest that variation within the 15q13-q14 chromosomal region, which encompasses an nAChR subunit, is associated with both schizophrenia and tobacco dependence.[110–114] These associations are potentially mediated by sensory gating deficits observed in individuals with schizophrenia;[115] nicotine normalises this deficit.[116] Given the strong association between schizophrenia and smoking, this is a promising area for future research.

Additional twin and family studies should be pursued first to determine the extent to which shared genetic liability contributes to the association.

3.4.2 Evidence from animal studies

In experimental animals, nicotine is reported to alleviate cognitive dysfunction, and it has been suggested that patients with schizophrenia may find this property of the drug particularly beneficial.[117,118] There is consistent evidence from animal studies that nicotine and tobacco smoking enhance pre-pulse inhibition, a form of sensorimotor gating, and attenuates the impairment in this measure observed in patients with schizophrenia.[119,120] Nicotine normalises schizophrenia-like deficits in sensorimotor gating induced by isolation rearing or the administration of amphetamine.[121] Impaired sensory gating has been linked to a reduction in the density of the α_7 subtype of the neuronal nicotinic receptor in the hippocampus, and with genetically linked polymorphisms in this receptor;[122,123] a recent postmortem study has shown that smoking selectively increases the expression and density of these receptors in the hippocampus of patients with schizophrenia.[110] Thus, the available data suggest that nicotine evokes this beneficial effect by both stimulating the receptors and enhancing their expression in the brains of patients with schizophrenia. Other studies in mice have shown that nicotine can reverse sensorimotor deficits evoked by the administration of a glutamate receptor antagonist, but that this response to nicotine is not observed in all strains of mice tested.[124] These data are consistent with the hypothesis that people who smoke may use nicotine as a form of self-medication but that its efficacy in this regard may depend on the interactions between nicotinic and glutamate receptors within the brain, which are genetically determined.

3.4.3 Evidence from human studies

Wing and colleagues[125] investigated cognitive performance variable among people with schizophrenia who both do and do not smoke. They found that non-smokers performed the poorest on measures of sustained attention, processing speed and response inhibition. Two experimental studies tested the hypothesis that nicotine can improve cognitive functioning in people with schizophrenia.[118,126] In a study by Depatie and colleagues,[126] nicotine patches improved the ability of participants to engage in tasks requiring sustained attention relative to placebo patches, findings that are consistent with research showing that people with schizophrenia have a diminished capacity to filter out irrelevant perceptual features of their environment, and that nicotine, through its action on inhibitory neurotransmission in the hippocampus, can correct this impairment.[116,127] The possibility that the beneficial effects of nicotine were related to the reversal of withdrawal could not be ruled out, however. Levin *et al*[117] were unable to demonstrate an effect of nicotine on selective attention in smokers with schizophrenia. Depatie and colleagues[126] suggest that differences in findings between these two studies may indicate that nicotine has differential effects on two different aspects of attention.

The great majority of people with schizophrenia begin smoking before the onset of psychosis.[128] Weiser and colleagues[129] investigated the hypothesis that future schizophrenia patients had higher rates of smoking before the manifestation of psychosis and the diagnosis and treatment of schizophrenia than non-psychiatric controls. Over 14,000 Israeli participants were recruited in late adolescence and followed an average of 10 years. These investigators found that the risk of developing schizophrenia during follow-up was twofold greater among smokers than non-smokers, and that among smokers this effect was exposure related. In a Swedish study of over 50,000 young adults, however, Zammit and colleagues[130] found that cigarette smoking was prospectively associated with a lower risk of developing schizophrenia. These investigators speculated that nicotine may have a modest neuroprotective effect for the development of schizophrenia, through nicotine effects on nAChRs and DA systems in the brain. A recent study, in which pre-morbid smoking was associated with later onset of schizophrenia, adds support to this interesting possibility;[131] relevant data are reviewed in more detail in Chapter 4. Individuals with schizophrenia appear to have an increased intensity of withdrawal symptoms during the first 2 weeks after a cessation attempt;[132] however, many outcome studies in which individuals with schizophrenia stop smoking do not find a long-term deterioration in schizophrenia symptoms or increased psychotic relapses.[107]

3.5 Attention deficit hyperactivity disorder

A link between ADHD and smoking has been documented repeatedly, even among adolescents with subclinical levels of ADHD characteristics.[133]

3.5.1 Evidence from genetic studies

The relationship between smoking and ADHD is complex, with maternal smoking during pregnancy long held to be a risk factor for offspring with ADHD.[134,135] It is possible that the relationship is confounded by a genetic correlation between maternal smoking and attentional/behavioural problems in the offspring. Furthermore, some twin studies have suggested that the association is less robust than previously thought;[136,137] however, such studies have not directly addressed whether the phenotypes are genetically or environmentally correlated in the offspring. Nevertheless, there are suggestions of a genetic correlation in the literature: one adolescent twin study reported high genetic, and moderate-to-high environmental, correlations between a general externalising liability factor and nicotine use,[138] although ADHD was not directly measured.

Few molecular genetic studies have explored the effects of specific genetic variants on both smoking/tobacco dependence and ADHD. However, evidence from a rat model of ADHD, which exhibits nicotinic receptor deficits relative to wild-type animals,[139] suggests that some such variants exist. Genome-wide association studies (GWAS) of ADHD have reported a modest association with variation (including duplications) in the human homologue of the same receptor subunit.[140,141] These findings are promising, and future work should utilise more global approaches (eg GWAS, twin studies) to explore additional shared genetic and environmental risk factors contributing to the phenotypic association. Although the precise nature of the relationship has yet to be untangled, clinicians should note that maternal smoking – particularly during pregnancy – and adolescent smoking are reasonably robust indicators of a liability to ADHD.

3.5.2 Evidence from animal studies

ADHD is routinely treated using drugs (eg methylphenidate and dexamphetamine) with stimulant properties, which resemble to some extent the psychopharmacological properties of nicotine. Smoking is more prevalent in patients with ADHD and it seems reasonable to suggest that patients with this condition may use tobacco as a form of self-medication. Although a number of authors have discussed their findings in the context of rationalising the putative role of ADHD in tobacco dependence, few studies have sought to explore the effects of nicotine in animal models of ADHD specifically. Studies with experimental rats and mice suggest that nicotine can improve sustained attention in some tasks such as the five-choice serial reaction time task (5CSRTT)[142–145] or a signal detection task.[146,147] In the latter task, nicotine also attenuates the deficit in attention evoked by the *N*-methyl-D-aspartate (NMDA) receptor antagonist dizolcipine.[148,149]

It has been suggested that the neurobiological mechanisms that underpin the ability of nicotine to improve attention and, especially, attenuate the impairment of attention may explain the vulnerability of patients with ADHD to nicotine/tobacco dependence.[118] Other studies have shown that nicotine improves attention and vigilance in performing the 5CSRTT in animals that exhibit less than optimal (<90% correct) performance, but may impair attention in animals with a good baseline performance (ie >90% correct).[150] This group also noted, however, that, in rats pre-treated with nicotine using a regimen designed to elicit sensitisation to the drug, nicotine evoked a significant increase in anticipatory responding which may be characteristic of disinhibition or impulsivity. Previous studies, using a different experimental paradigm, also suggest that repeated or chronic nicotine elicits disinhibition in experimental rats.[151,152] Thus, in studies with experimental animals, nicotine, although having some psychopharmacological characteristics of an anti-ADHD agent, does not seem to have all the properties necessary to alleviate all the symptoms of the condition.

3.5.3 Evidence from human studies

Studies have supported the hypothesis that nicotine improves cognitive functions in people with ADHD,[153–157] eg Gehricke and colleagues[156] found an effect of nicotine relative to placebo patch on attention and concentration in young adults with ADHD who smoked. Smokers wore a nicotine patch for 2 days and a placebo patch for 2 days, and used electronic diaries to record ADHD symptoms during their normal daily routines. However, it is difficult to distinguish direct effects of nicotine versus withdrawal relief due to nicotine administration in studies such as this where people who smoke regularly are asked to abstain from smoking. Therefore, using a similar design, Gehricke and colleagues[155] investigated the effects of nicotine in young adults with ADHD who both did and did not smoke. They found that nicotine patches improved attention and reduced difficulty concentrating compared with placebo patch in smokers with ADHD. Critically, they found almost identical results for non-smokers. As noted above, studies of the effect of nicotine in non-smokers are important to distinguish between attentional effects resulting from reversal of cognitively based nicotine withdrawal effects (eg impaired concentration) and any beneficial effects that are independent of the reversal of withdrawal symptoms. In their laboratory study investigating the effects of nicotine on ADHD symptoms, Levin and colleagues[157] found that nicotine versus placebo patch enhanced attention in both smokers and non-smokers (the effect was greater in non-smokers); concentration was enhanced only in smokers. Similar effects for nicotine versus placebo on cognitive functioning were found in a study of non-smokers with ADHD.[93] By contrast, Conners and colleagues[154] found an effect for smokers but not non-smokers. Nicotine has also been found to beneficially affect behavioural disinhibition and other symptoms of ADHD,[158] although the results have been inconsistent.[153]

In a 4-year prospective study of adolescents, Milberger and colleagues[159] found that ADHD symptoms were significantly related to smoking initiation; at follow-up, 19% of participants with ADHD had initiated smoking versus 11% without ADHD. In addition, participants with ADHD had an earlier age of onset: 71% of smokers with ADHD began smoking before age 17 compared with 27% of smokers without ADHD. Smoking initiation was also significantly related to psychiatric co-morbidity. The prevalence of cigarette smoking was 10% among participants with ADHD only and 27% in participants with one or more additional psychiatric disorder (eg conduct disorder, anxiety disorder). However, the association between ADHD and smoking initiation remained significant after the influence of co-morbidities was statistically controlled. Fuemmeler and colleagues[133] also found that ADHD symptoms were associated with smoking initiation and progression to regular use. Interestingly, however, when these investigators assessed the separate effects of inattentive and impulsive–hyperactive symptoms, only the latter were significantly associated with initiation and progression. Whalen and colleagues[160] found that adolescents with untreated ADHD were more likely to initiate smoking than their counterparts who were receiving medication. In addition, they smoked more regularly.[161] Finally, smokers with ADHD appear to be at risk for severe tobacco dependence.[162]

The impairments in attention and concentration characteristic of ADHD are frequently associated with problems in affect regulation and arousal, including depression-impaired anger management.[163,164] In a study described above, Gehricke and colleagues[155] investigated the mood effects of nicotine in adults with ADHD. Although differences were modest, participants reported lower levels of negative affect (nervousness, stress, anger) in the nicotine versus placebo patch condition. Similar between-patch differences were found in both smokers and non-smokers. Bekker and colleagues[153] reported similar results in smokers with ADHD. Small improvements in the mood of non-smokers with ADHD after nicotine versus placebo administration have been observed in other studies.[154,157]

3.6 Smoking and dementia

Apolipoprotein E genotype has been reported to modify the effect of some exposures for dementia; however, its role as a risk factor for smoking remains controversial, with one large study suggesting stronger associations between smoking and incident dementia in the absence of the ε4 allele,[165] another finding stronger associations in the presence of this allele[166] and a third finding no difference between these strata.[167] Finally, the impact of improving a variety of lifestyles on risk of dementia was recently modelled and it was estimated that each 5% reduction in smoking prevalence would result in a 2% reduction in dementia risk.[168] In terms of potential underlying mechanisms, associations have been reported between smoking and neuritic plaques in a neuropathological follow-up study nested within a large cohort,[167] suggesting direct influences on Alzheimer's disease progression. However, the effect of smoking on cerebral perfusion[169] and cerebrovascular disease in general is also likely to be important.

Understanding of the relationship between smoking and dementia risk has changed dramatically over recent decades, from early suggestions of a protective effect to later confirmation as a risk factor. Meta-analyses have found an association between dementia risk and current smoking,[170,171] but no association with former smoking.[170,171] One recent study has also reported an association between passive smoking and increased dementia risk,[172] with supporting evidence of associations between passive smoking and cognitive impairment.[173] This evidence is reviewed further in Chapter 4.

3.7 Future studies

Ultimately, observational data do not provide unequivocal evidence of causation, and experimental studies to elicit further detail are either not possible in clinical populations or unethical. Mendelian randomisation,[174] whereby genetic information can be used to test causal hypotheses regarding the effects of environmental exposures such as cigarette smoking, may allow a better understanding of the causal relationship between smoking and mental health. This requires specific polymorphisms that have been shown to be robustly associated with measures of exposure (eg number of cigarettes per day). Given the random assortment of genes from parents to offspring that occurs during gamete formation and conception, genotype should not be related to potential confounders (although confounding may still occur, eg due to linkage disequilibrium with other loci, or pleiotropic effects whereby single genetic loci are associated with multiple phenotypes). Therefore, a robust genetic influence on smoking would be akin to a randomised trial where individuals are effectively assigned to a high or low smoking exposure group, and could be used to test the causal relationship between smoking and depression. A number of loci have recently emerged that are convincingly associated with smoking.[175] These might, in principle, be used to address questions of causation regarding the effects of cigarette smoking.[101,176]

3.8 Summary

> - Although smoking, and high levels of dependence on smoking, are both more common in people with mental disorders, the mechanisms underlying these associations are uncertain.
> - There is some evidence of common genetic determinants of both smoking and specific mental disorders, particularly depression and schizophrenia.
> - Experimental evidence suggests that nicotine can relieve symptoms of anxiety, depression, schizophrenia and ADHD, although nicotine withdrawal symptoms may then exacerbate symptoms of mental disorders.
> - People with some mental disorders may use nicotine to ameliorate symptoms such as depression or anxiety (the self-medication model).
> - However, the symptoms of mental disorders can be confused with or exacerbated by those of nicotine withdrawal, hence resulting in false attribution of relief to effects on mental disorders.
> - The effects of constituents of tobacco and tobacco smoke other than nicotine on mood and cognition remain unclear.

> The association between smoking and mental disorders is therefore complex and further work is needed to help improve understanding.

References

1 Corrigall WA, Coen KM. Nicotine maintains robust self-administration in rats on a limited-access schedule. *Psychopharmacology* 1989;99:473–8.
2 Donny EC, Caggiula AR, Knopf S, Brown C. Nicotine self-administration in rats. *Psychopharmacology* 1995;122:390–94.
3 Epping-Jordan MP, Watkins SS, Koob GF, Markou A. Dramatic decreases in brain reward function during nicotine withdrawal. *Nature* 1998;393:76–9.
4 Malin DH, Lake JR, Newlin-Maultsby P, *et al*. Rodent model of nicotine abstinence syndrome. *Pharmacology, Biochemistry and Behavior* 1992;43:779–84.
5 Kenny PJ, Markou A. Neurobiology of the nicotine withdrawal syndrome. *Pharmacology, Biochemistry and Behavior* 2001;70:531–49.
6 Malin DH, Goyarzu P. Rodent models of nicotine withdrawal syndrome. *Handbook of Experimental Pharmacology* 2009;192:401–34.
7 Di Chiara G. Role of dopamine in the behavioural actions of nicotine related to addiction. *European Journal of Pharmacology* 2000;393:295–314.
8 Di Chiara G, Bassareo V, Fenu S, *et al*. Dopamine and drug addiction: the nucleus accumbens shell connection. *Neuropharmacology* 2004;47(suppl 1):227–41.
9 Lecca D, Cacciapaglia F, Valentini V, *et al*. Preferential increase of extracellular dopamine in the rat nucleus accumbens shell as compared to that in the core during acquisition and maintenance of intravenous nicotine self-administration. *Psychopharmacology* 2006;184:435–46.
10 Benwell ME, Balfour DJ. The effects of acute and repeated nicotine treatment on nucleus accumbens dopamine and locomotor activity. *British Journal of Pharmacology* 1992;105:849–56.
11 Cadoni C, Di Chiara G. Differential changes in accumbens shell and core dopamine in behavioral sensitization to nicotine. *European Journal of Pharmacology* 2000;387:R23–5.
12 Iyaniwura TT, Wright AE, Balfour DJ. Evidence that mesoaccumbens dopamine and locomotor responses to nicotine in the rat are influenced by pretreatment dose and strain. *Psychopharmacology* 2001;158:73–9.
13 Di Chiara G. A motivational learning hypothesis of the role of mesolimbic dopamine in compulsive drug use. *Journal of Psychopharmacology* 1998;12:54–67.
14 Di Chiara G, Bassareo V. Reward system and addiction: what dopamine does and doesn't do. *Current Opinion in Pharmacology* 2007;7:69–76.
15 Balfour DJ. The neuronal pathways mediating the behavioral and addictive properties of nicotine. *Handbook of Experimental Pharmacology* 2009;192:209–33.
16 Fowler JS, Logan J, Wang GJ, Volkow ND. Monoamine oxidase and cigarette smoking. *Neurotoxicology* 2003;24:75–82.
17 Fowler JS, Volkow ND, Wang GJ, *et al*. Inhibition of monoamine oxidase B in the brains of smokers. *Nature* 1996;379:733–6.
18 Fowler JS, Volkow ND, Wang GJ, *et al*. Brain monoamine oxidase A inhibition in cigarette smokers. *Proceedings of the National Academy of Sciences of the USA* 1996;93:14065–9.
19 Guillem K, Vouillac C, Azar MR, *et al*. Monoamine oxidase inhibition dramatically increases the motivation to self-administer nicotine in rats. *Journal of Neuroscience* 2005;25:8593–600.

20 Guillem K, Vouillac C, Azar MR, et al. Monoamine oxidase A rather than monoamine oxidase B inhibition increases nicotine reinforcement in rats. *European Journal of Neuroscience* 2006;24:3532–40.

21 Villegier AS, Lotfipour S, McQuown SC, Belluzzi JD, Leslie FM. Tranylcypromine enhancement of nicotine self-administration. *Neuropharmacology* 2007;52:1415–25.

22 Caggiula AR, Donny EC, Chaudhri N, et al.. Importance of nonpharmacological factors in nicotine self-administration. *Physiology and Behavior* 2002;77:683–7.

23 Caggiula AR, Donny EC, White AR, et al. Cue dependency of nicotine self-administration and smoking. *Pharmacology, Biochemistry and Behavior* 2001;70:515–30.

24 Chaudhri N, Caggiula AR, Donny EC, et al. Complex interactions between nicotine and nonpharmacological stimuli reveal multiple roles for nicotine in reinforcement. *Psychopharmacology* 2006;184:353–66.

25 Rose JE, Behm FM, Westman EC, Johnson M. Dissociating nicotine and nonnicotine components of cigarette smoking. *Pharmacology, Biochemistry and Behavior* 2000;67:71–81.

26 Brauer LH, Behm FM, Lane JD, et al. Individual differences in smoking reward from de-nicotinized cigarettes. *Nicotine and Tobacco Research* 2001;3:101–9.

27 Rose JE. Nicotine and nonnicotine factors in cigarette addiction. *Psychopharmacology* 2006;184:274–85.

28 Caggiula AR, Donny EC, Palmatier MI, Liu X, Chaudhri N, Sved AF. The role of nicotine in smoking: a dual-reinforcement model. *Nebraska Symposium on Motivation* 2009;55:91–109.

29 Khantzian EJ. The self-medication hypothesis of substance use disorders: a reconsideration and recent applications. *Harvard Review of Psychiatry* 1997;4:231–44.

30 Markou A, Kosten TR, Koob GF. Neurobiological similarities in depression and drug dependence: a self-medication hypothesis. *Neuropsychopharmacology* 1998;18:135–74.

31 Amitai N, Markou A. Increased impulsivity and disrupted attention induced by repeated phencyclidine are not attenuated by chronic quetiapine treatment. *Pharmacology, Biochemistry and Behavior* 2009;93:248–57.

32 Picciotto MR, Brunzell DH, Caldarone BJ. Effect of nicotine and nicotinic receptors on anxiety and depression. *NeuroReport* 2002;13:1097–106.

33 Watkins SS, Koob GF, Markou A. Neural mechanisms underlying nicotine addiction: acute positive reinforcement and withdrawal. *Nicotine and Tobacco Research* 2000;2:19–37.

34 Dursun SM, Kutcher S. Smoking, nicotine and psychiatric disorders: evidence for therapeutic role, controversies and implications for future research. *Medical Hypotheses* 1999;52:101–9.

35 Mihailescu S, Drucker-Colin R. Nicotine, brain nicotinic receptors, and neuropsychiatric disorders. *Archives of Medical Research* 2000;31:131–44.

36 Ferguson SM, Brodkin JD, Lloyd GK, Menzaghi F. Antidepressant-like effects of the subtype-selective nicotinic acetylcholine receptor agonist, SIB-1508Y, in the learned helplessness rat model of depression. *Psychopharmacology* 2000;152:295–303.

37 Tizabi Y, Overstreet DH, Rezvani AH, et al. Antidepressant effects of nicotine in an animal model of depression. *Psychopharmacology* 1999;142:193–9.

38 Balfour DJ, Ridley DL. The effects of nicotine on neural pathways implicated in depression: a factor in nicotine addiction? *Pharmacology, Biochemistry and Behavior* 2000;66:79–85.

39 Kapur S, Mann JJ. Role of the dopaminergic system in depression. *Biological Psychiatry* 1992;32(1):1–17.

40 Porcu P, Sogliano C, Cinus M, et al. Nicotine-induced changes in cerebrocortical neuroactive steroids and plasma corticosterone concentrations in the rat. *Pharmacology, Biochemistry and Behavior* 2003;74:683–90.

41 Rudehill A, Franco-Cereceda A, Hemsen A, et al. Cigarette smoke-induced elevation of plasma neuropeptide Y levels in man. *Clinical Physiology* 1989;9:243–8.

42 Hahn B, Sharples CG, Wonnacott S, Shoaib M, Stolerman IP. Attentional effects of nicotinic agonists in rats. *Neuropharmacology* 2003;44:1054–67.

43 Picciotto MR, Caldarone BJ, King SL, Zachariou V. Nicotinic receptors in the brain. Links between molecular biology and behavior. *Neuropsychopharmacology* 2000;22:451–65.

44 Yamazaki Y, Hamaue N, Sumikawa K. Nicotine compensates for the loss of cholinergic function to enhance long-term potentiation induction. *Brain Research* 2002;946(1):148–52.

45 Martin LF, Kem WR, Freedman R. Alpha-7 nicotinic receptor agonists: potential new candidates for the treatment of schizophrenia. *Psychopharmacology* 2004;174:54–64.

46 Dalack GW, Healy DJ, Meador-Woodruff JH. Nicotine dependence in schizophrenia: clinical phenomena and laboratory findings. *American Journal of Psychiatry* 1998;155:1490–501.

47 Chassin L, Presson C, Seo DC, et al. Multiple trajectories of cigarette smoking and the intergenerational transmission of smoking: a multigenerational, longitudinal study of a Midwestern community sample. *Health Psychology* 2008;27:819–28.

48 Mayhew KP, Flay BR, Mott JA. Stages in the development of adolescent smoking. *Drug and Alcohol Dependence* 2000;59(suppl 1):S61–81.

49 Kendler KS, Neale MC, MacLean CJ, et al. Smoking and major depression. A causal analysis. *Archives of General Psychiatry* 1993;50:36–43.

50 Korhonen T, Broms U, Varjonen J, et al. Smoking behaviour as a predictor of depression among Finnish men and women: a prospective cohort study of adult twins. *Psychological Medicine* 2007;37:705–15.

51 Lyons M, Hitsman B, Xian H, et al. A twin study of smoking, nicotine dependence, and major depression in men. *Nicotine and Tobacco Research* 2008;10:97–108.

52 Edwards AC, Maes HH, Pedersen NL, Kendler KS. A population-based twin study of the genetic and environmental relationship of major depression, regular tobacco use and nicotine dependence. *Psychological Medicine* 2011;41:395–405.

53 Lajtha A, Sershen H. Nicotine: alcohol reward interactions. *Neurochemical Research* 2010;35:1248–58.

54 Andreasen JT, Redrobe JP. Antidepressant-like effects of nicotine and mecamylamine in the mouse forced swim and tail suspension tests: role of strain, test and sex. *Behavioral Pharmacology* 2009;20:286–95.

55 Suemaru K, Yasuda K, Cui R, et al. Antidepressant-like action of nicotine in forced swimming test and brain serotonin in mice. *Physiology and Behavior* 2006;88:545–9.

56 Vazquez-Palacios G, Bonilla-Jaime H, Velazquez-Moctezuma J. Antidepressant-like effects of the acute and chronic administration of nicotine in the rat forced swimming test and its interaction with fluoxetine [correction of flouxetine]. *Pharmacology, Biochemistry and Behavior* 2004;78:165–9.

57 Djuric VJ, Dunn E, Overstreet DH, Dragomir A, Steiner M. Antidepressant effect of ingested nicotine in female rats of Flinders resistant and sensitive lines. *Physiology and Behavior* 1999;67:533–7.

58 Tizabi Y, Getachew B, Rezvani AH, Hauser SR, Overstreet DH. Antidepressant-like effects of nicotine and reduced nicotinic receptor binding in the Fawn-Hooded rat, an animal model of co-morbid depression and alcoholism. *Progress in Neuro-Psychopharmacology and Biological Psychiatry* 2009;33:398–402.

59 Vieyra-Reyes P, Mineur YS, Picciotto MR, et al. Antidepressant-like effects of nicotine and transcranial magnetic stimulation in the olfactory bulbectomy rat model of depression. *Brain Research Bulletin* 2008;77:13–8.

60 Andreasen JT, Henningsen K, Bate S, Christiansen S, Wiborg O. Nicotine reverses anhedonic-like response and cognitive impairment in the rat chronic mild stress model of depression: comparison with sertraline. *Journal of Psychopharmacology* 2010;25:1134–41.

61 Tronci V, Balfour DJ. The effects of the mGluR5 receptor antagonist 6-methyl-2-(phenylethynyl)-pyridine (MPEP) on the stimulation of dopamine release evoked by nicotine in the rat brain. *Behavioural Brain Research* 2011;219:354–7.

62 Palmatier MI, Liu X, Caggiula AR, Donny EC, Sved AF. The role of nicotinic acetylcholine receptors in the primary reinforcing and reinforcement-enhancing effects of nicotine. *Neuropsychopharmacology* 2007;32:1098–108.

63 Palmatier MI, Matteson GL, Black JJ, et al. The reinforcement enhancing effects of nicotine depend on the incentive value of non-drug reinforcers and increase with repeated drug injections. *Drug and Alcohol Dependence* 2007;89:52–9.

64 Bozarth MA, Pudiak CM, KuoLee R. Effect of chronic nicotine on brain stimulation reward. I. Effect of daily injections. *Behavioural Brain Research* 1998;96:185–8.

65 Clarke PB, Kumar R. Effects of nicotine and d-amphetamine on intracranial self-stimulation in a shuttle box test in rats. *Psychopharmacology* 1984;84:109–14.

66 Kenny PJ, Markou A. Nicotine self-administration acutely activates brain reward systems and induces a long-lasting increase in reward sensitivity. *Neuropsychopharmacology* 2006;31:1203–11.

67 Nestler EJ, Carlezon WA, Jr. The mesolimbic dopamine reward circuit in depression. *Biological Psychiatry* 2006;59:1151–9.

68 Paterson NE, Markou A. Animal models and treatments for addiction and depression co-morbidity. *Neurotoxin Research* 2007;11:1–32.

69 Benwell ME, Balfour DJ, Khadra LF. Studies on the influence of nicotine infusions on mesolimbic dopamine and locomotor responses to nicotine. *Clinical Investigations* 1994;72:233–9.

70 Turner JR, Castellano LM, Blendy JA. Nicotinic partial agonists varenicline and sazetidine-A have differential effects on affective behavior. *Journal of Pharmacology and Experimental Therapeutics* 2010;334:665–72.

71 Mineur YS, Picciotto MR. Nicotine receptors and depression: revisiting and revising the cholinergic hypothesis. *Trends in Pharmacological Science* 2010;31:580–6.

72 Simon NM. Generalized anxiety disorder and psychiatric comorbidities such as depression, bipolar disorder, and substance abuse. *Journal of Clinical Psychiatry* 2009;70(suppl 2):10–4.

73 Brioni JD, O'Neill AB, Kim DJ, et al. Anxiolytic-like effects of the novel cholinergic channel activator ABT-418. *Journal of Pharmacology and Experimental Therapeutics* 1994;271:353–61.

74 Turner JR, Castellano LM, Blendy JA. Parallel anxiolytic-like effects and upregulation of neuronal nicotinic acetylcholine receptors following chronic nicotine and varenicline. *Nicotine and Tobacco Research* 2010;13:41–6.

75 Vale AL, Green S. Effects of chlordiazepoxide, nicotine and *d*-amphetamine in the rat potentiated startle model of anxiety. *Behavioural Pharmacology* 1996;7:138–43.

76 Balfour DJ, Graham CA, Vale AL. Studies on the possible role of brain 5-HT systems and adrenocortical activity in behavioural responses to nicotine and diazepam in an elevated X-maze. *Psychopharmacology* 1986;90:528–32.

77 Caldarone BJ, King SL, Picciotto MR. Sex differences in anxiety-like behavior and locomotor activity following chronic nicotine exposure in mice. *Neuroscience Letters* 2008;439:187–91.

78 Ouagazzal AM, Kenny PJ, File SE. Modulation of behaviour on trials 1 and 2 in the elevated plus-maze test of anxiety after systemic and hippocampal administration of nicotine. *Psychopharmacology* 1999;144:54–60.

79 Biala G, Budzynska B. Effects of acute and chronic nicotine on elevated plus maze in mice: involvement of calcium channels. *Life Sciences* 2006 30;79:81–8.

80 Benwell ME, Balfour DJ. Effects of nicotine administration and its withdrawal on plasma corticosterone and brain 5-hydroxyindoles. *Psychopharmacology* 1979;63:7–11.

81 Buczek Y, Le AD, Wang A, Stewart J, Shaham Y. Stress reinstates nicotine seeking but not sucrose solution seeking in rats. *Psychopharmacology* 1999;144:183–8.

82 Martin-Garcia E, Barbano MF, Galeote L, Maldonado R. New operant model of nicotine-seeking behaviour in mice. *International Journal of Neuropsychopharmacology* 2009;12:343–56.

83 Jonkman S, Risbrough VB, Geyer MA, Markou A. Spontaneous nicotine withdrawal potentiates the effects of stress in rats. *Neuropsychopharmacology* 2008;33:2131–8.

84 O'Dell LE, Khroyan TV. Rodent models of nicotine reward: what do they tell us about tobacco abuse in humans? *Pharmacology, Biochemistry and Behavior* 2009;91:481–8.

85 Kalman D. The subjective effects of nicotine: methodological issues, a review of experimental studies, and recommendations for future research. *Nicotine and Tobacco Research* 2002;4:25–70.

86 Kalman D, Smith SS. Does nicotine do what we think it does? A meta-analytic review of the subjective effects of nicotine in nasal spray and intravenous studies with smokers and nonsmokers. *Nicotine and Tobacco Research* 2005;7:317–33.

87 Salin-Pascual RJ, de la Fuente JR, Galicia-Polo L, Drucker-Colin R. Effects of transderman nicotine on mood and sleep in nonsmoking major depressed patients. *Psychopharmacology* 1995;121:476–9.

88 Salin-Pascual RJ, Drucker-Colin R. A novel effect of nicotine on mood and sleep in major depression. *NeuroReport* 1998;9:57–60.

89 Salin-Pascual RJ, Rosas M, Jimenez-Genchi A, Rivera-Meza BL, Delgado-Parra V. Antidepressant effect of transdermal nicotine patches in nonsmoking patients with major depression. *Journal of Clinical Psychiatry* 1996;57:387–9.

90 Cox LS, Patten CA, Krahn LE, et al. The effect of nicotine patch therapy on depression in nonsmokers: a preliminary study. *Journal of Addictive Disease* 2003;22:75–85.

91 McClernon FJ, Hiott FB, Westman EC, Rose JE, Levin ED. Transdermal nicotine attenuates depression symptoms in nonsmokers: a double-blind, placebo-controlled trial. *Psychopharmacology* 2006;189:125–33.

92 Gilbert DG, Robinson JH, Chamberlin CL, Spielberger CD. Effects of smoking/nicotine on anxiety, heart rate, and lateralization of EEG during a stressful movie. *Psychophysiology* 1989;26:311–20.

93 Levin ED, Conners CK, Silva D, Canu W, March J. Effects of chronic nicotine and methylphenidate in adults with attention deficit/hyperactivity disorder. *Experimental and Clinical Psychopharmacology* 2001;9:83–90.

94 Jamner LD, Shapiro D, Jarvik ME. Nicotine reduces the frequency of anger reports in smokers and nonsmokers with high but not low hostility: an ambulatory study. *Experimental and Clinical Psychopharmacology* 1999;7:454–63.

95 Kassel JD, Unrod M. Smoking, anxiety, and attention: support for the role of nicotine in attentionally mediated anxiolysis. *Journal of Abnormal Psychology* 2000;109:161–6.

96 Audrain-McGovern J, Rodriguez D, Kassel JD. Adolescent smoking and depression: evidence for self-medication and peer smoking mediation. *Addiction* 2009;104:1743–56.

97 Fergusson DM, Goodwin RD, Horwood LJ. Major depression and cigarette smoking: results of a 21-year longitudinal study. *Psychological Medicine* 2003;33:1357–67.

98 Killen JD, Robinson TN, Haydel KF, *et al*. Prospective study of risk factors for the initiation of cigarette smoking. *Journal of Consulting and Clinical Psychology* 1997;65:1011–6.

99 Patton GC, Carlin JB, Coffey C, *et al*. Depression, anxiety, and smoking initiation: a prospective study over 3 years. *American Journal of Public Health* 1998;88:1518–22.

100 Kobus K. Peers and adolescent smoking. *Addiction* 2003;98(suppl 1):37–55.

101 Munafo MR, Araya R. Cigarette smoking and depression: a question of causation. *British Journal of Psychiatry* 2011;196:425–6.

102 Wang MQ, Fitzhugh EC, Green BL, *et al*. Prospective social-psychological factors of adolescent smoking progression. *Journal of Adolescent Health* 1999;24:2–9.

103 Whalen CK, Jamner LD, Henker B, Delfino RJ. Smoking and moods in adolescents with depressive and aggressive dispositions: evidence from surveys and electronic diaries. *Health Psychology* 2001;20:99–111.

104 Breslau N, Kilbey MM, Andreski P. Nicotine dependence and major depression. New evidence from a prospective investigation. *Archives of General Psychiatry* 1993;50:31–5.

105 McKenzie M, Olsson CA, Jorm AF, Romaniuk H, Patton GC. Association of adolescent symptoms of depression and anxiety with daily smoking and nicotine dependence in young adulthood: findings from a 10-year longitudinal study. *Addiction* 2010;105:1652–9.

106 Karp I, O'Loughlin J, Hanley J, Tyndale RF, Paradis G. Risk factors for tobacco dependence in adolescent smokers. *Tobacco Control* 2006;15:199–204.

107 Ziedonis D, Hitsman B, Beckham JC, *et al*. Tobacco use and cessation in psychiatric disorders: National Institute of Mental Health report. *Nicotine and Tobacco Research* 2008;10:1691–715.

108 Hitsman B, Borrelli B, McChargue DE, Spring B, Niaura R. History of depression and smoking cessation outcome: a meta-analysis. *Journal of Consulting and Clinical Psychology* 2003;71:657–63.

109 Lyons MJ, Bar JL, Kremen WS, *et al*. Nicotine and familial vulnerability to schizophrenia: a discordant twin study. *Journal of Abnormal Psychology* 2002;111:687–93.

110 Mexal S, Berger R, Logel J, Ross *et al*. Differential regulation of alpha7 nicotinic receptor gene (CHRNA7) expression in schizophrenic smokers. *Journal of Molecular Neuroscience* 2010;40:185–95.

111 Riley BP, Makoff A, Mogudi-Carter M, *et al*. Haplotype transmission disequilibrium and evidence for linkage of the CHRNA7 gene region to schizophrenia in Southern African Bantu families. *American Journal of Medical Genetics* 2000;96:196–201.

112 Saccone NL, Schwantes-An TH, Wang JC, *et al*. Multiple cholinergic nicotinic receptor genes affect nicotine dependence risk in African and European Americans. *Genes and Brain Behaviour* 2010;9:741–50.

113 Stephens SH, Franks A, Berger R, *et al*. Multiple genes in the 15q13-q14 chromosomal region are associated with schizophrenia. *Psychiatric Genetics* 2012;22:1–14.

114 Tsuang DW, Skol AD, Faraone SV, *et al*. Examination of genetic linkage of chromosome 15 to schizophrenia in a large Veterans Affairs Cooperative Study sample. *American Journal of Medical Genetics* 2001;105:662–8.

115 Clementz BA, Geyer MA, Braff DL. P50 suppression among schizophrenia and normal comparison subjects: a methodological analysis. *Biological Psychiatry* 1997;41:1035–44.

116 Adler LE, Hoffer LD, Wiser A, Freedman R. Normalization of auditory physiology by cigarette smoking in schizophrenic patients. *American Journal of Psychiatry* 1993;150:1856–61.

117 Levin ED, McClernon FJ, Rezvani AH. Nicotinic effects on cognitive function: behavioral characterization, pharmacological specification, and anatomic localization. *Psychopharmacology* 2006;184:523–39.

118 Levin ED, Rezvani AH. Nicotinic treatment for cognitive dysfunction. *Current Drug Targets CNS Neurological Disorders* 2002;1:423–31.

119 Braff DL, Geyer MA, Swerdlow NR. Human studies of prepulse inhibition of startle: normal subjects, patient groups, and pharmacological studies. *Psychopharmacology* 2001;156:234–58.

120 Kumari V, Soni W, Sharma T. Influence of cigarette smoking on prepulse inhibition of the acoustic startle response in schizophrenia. *Human Psychopharmacology* 2001;16:321–6.

121 Stevens KE, Wear KD. Normalizing effects of nicotine and a novel nicotinic agonist on hippocampal auditory gating in two animal models. *Pharmacology, Biochemistry and Behaviour* 1997;57:869–74.

122 Freedman R, Olincy A, Ross RG, *et al*. The genetics of sensory gating deficits in schizophrenia. *Current Psychiatry Report* 2003;5:155–61.

123 Leonard S, Adler LE, Benhammou K, *et al*. Smoking and mental illness. *Pharmacology, Biochemistry and Behaviour* 2001;70:561–70.

124 Spielewoy C, Markou A. Strain-specificity in nicotine attenuation of phencyclidine-induced disruption of prepulse inhibition in mice: relevance to smoking in schizophrenia patients. *Behavior Genetics* 2004;34:343–54.

125 Wing VC, Bacher I, Sacco KA, George TP. Neuropsychological performance in patients with schizophrenia and controls as a function of cigarette smoking status. *Psychiatry Research* 2011;188:320–6.

126 Depatie L, O'Driscoll GA, Holahan AL, *et al*. Nicotine and behavioral markers of risk for schizophrenia: a double-blind, placebo-controlled, cross-over study. *Neuropsychopharmacology* 2002;27:1056–70.

127 Adler LE, Olincy A, Waldo M, *et al*. Schizophrenia, sensory gating, and nicotinic receptors. *Schizophrenia Bulletin* 1998;24:189–202.

128 Kelly C, McCreadie RG. Smoking habits, current symptoms, and premorbid characteristics of schizophrenic patients in Nithsdale, Scotland. *American Journal of Psychiatry* 1999;156:1751–7.

129 Weiser M, Reichenberg A, Grotto I, *et al*. Higher rates of cigarette smoking in male adolescents before the onset of schizophrenia: a historical-prospective cohort study. *American Journal of Psychiatry* 2004;161:1219–23.

130 Zammit S, Allebeck P, Dalman C, *et al*. Investigating the association between cigarette smoking and schizophrenia in a cohort study. *American Journal of Psychiatry* 2003;160:2216–21.

131 Ma X, Li C, Meng H, *et al*. Premorbid tobacco smoking is associated with later age at onset in schizophrenia. *Psychiatry Research* 2010;178:461–6.

132 George TP, Vessicchio JC, Termine A, *et al*. Effects of smoking abstinence on visuospatial working memory function in schizophrenia. *Neuropsychopharmacology* 2002;26:75–85.

133 Fuemmeler BF, Kollins SH, McClernon FJ. Attention deficit hyperactivity disorder symptoms predict nicotine dependence and progression to regular smoking from adolescence to young adulthood. *Journal of Pediatric Psychology* 2007;32:1203–13.

134 Milberger S, Biederman J, Faraone SV, Chen L, Jones J. Is maternal smoking during pregnancy a risk factor for attention deficit hyperactivity disorder in children? *American Journal of Psychiatry* 1996;153:1138–42.

135 Thapar A, Fowler T, Rice F, et al. Maternal smoking during pregnancy and attention deficit hyperactivity disorder symptoms in offspring. *American Journal of Psychiatry* 2003;160:1985–9.

136 D'Onofrio BM, Van Hulle CA, Waldman ID, et al. Smoking during pregnancy and offspring externalizing problems: an exploration of genetic and environmental confounds. *Developmental Psychopathology* 2008;20:139–64.

137 Knopik VS, Sparrow EP, Madden PA, et al. Contributions of parental alcoholism, prenatal substance exposure, and genetic transmission to child ADHD risk: a female twin study. *Psychological Medicine* 2005;35:625–35.

138 Hicks BM, Schalet BD, Malone SM, Iacono WG, McGue M. Psychometric and genetic architecture of substance use disorder and behavioral disinhibition measures for gene association studies. *Behavior Genetics* 2010;41:459–75.

139 Wigestrand MB, Mineur YS, Heath CJ, et al. Decreased alpha4beta2 nicotinic receptor number in the absence of mRNA changes suggests post-transcriptional regulation in the spontaneously hypertensive rat model of ADHD. *Journal of Neurochemistry* 2011;119:240–50.

140 Stergiakouli E, Hamshere M, Holmans P, et al. Investigating the contribution of common genetic variants to the risk and pathogenesis of ADHD. *American Journal of Psychiatry* 2011;169:186–194.

141 Williams NM, Franke B, Mick E, et al. Genome-wide analysis of copy number variants in attention deficit hyperactivity disorder: the role of rare variants and duplications at 15q13.3. *American Journal of Psychiatry* 2012;169:195–204.

142 Hahn B, Shoaib M, Stolerman IP. Nicotine-induced enhancement of attention in the five-choice serial reaction time task: the influence of task demands. *Psychopharmacology* 2002;162:129–37.

143 Hahn B, Stolerman IP. Nicotine-induced attentional enhancement in rats: effects of chronic exposure to nicotine. *Neuropsychopharmacology* 2002;27:712–22.

144 Mirza NR, Bright JL. Nicotine-induced enhancements in the five-choice serial reaction time task in rats are strain-dependent. *Psychopharmacology* 2001;154:8–12.

145 Mirza NR, Stolerman IP. Nicotine enhances sustained attention in the rat under specific task conditions. *Psychopharmacology* 1998;138:266–74.

146 Rezvani AH, Bushnell PJ, Levin ED. Effects of nicotine and mecamylamine on choice accuracy in an operant visual signal detection task in female rats. *Psychopharmacology* 2002;164:369–75.

147 Rezvani AH, Caldwell DP, Levin ED. Chronic nicotine interactions with clozapine and risperidone and attentional function in rats. *Progress in Neuro-Psychopharmacology and Biological Psychiatry* 2006;30:190–7.

148 Rezvani AH, Kholdebarin E, Dawson E, Levin ED. Nicotine and clozapine effects on attentional performance impaired by the NMDA antagonist dizocilpine in female rats. *Int Journal of Neuropsychopharmacology* 2008;11:63–70.

149 Rezvani AH, Levin ED. Nicotinic-glutamatergic interactions and attentional performance on an operant visual signal detection task in female rats. *European Journal of Pharmacology* 2003;465:83–90.

150 Day M, Pan JB, Buckley MJ, et al. Differential effects of ciproxifan and nicotine on impulsivity and attention measures in the 5-choice serial reaction time test. *Biochemical Pharmacology* 2007;73:1123–34.

151 Ericson M, Olausson P, Engel JA, Soderpalm B. Nicotine induces disinhibitory behavior in the rat after subchronic peripheral nicotinic acetylcholine receptor blockade. *European Journal of Pharmacology* 2000;397:103–11.

152 Olausson P, Engel JA, Soderpalm B. Behavioral sensitization to nicotine is associated with behavioral disinhibition; counteraction by citalopram. *Psychopharmacology* 1999;142:111–19.

153 Bekker EM, Bocker KB, Van Hunsel F, van den Berg MC, Kenemans JL. Acute effects of nicotine on attention and response inhibition. *Pharmacology, Biochemistry and Behavior* 2005;82:539–48.

154 Conners CK, Levin ED, Sparrow E, *et al*. Nicotine and attention in adult attention deficit hyperactivity disorder (ADHD). *Psychopharmacology Bulletin* 1996;32:67–73.

155 Gehricke JG, Hong N, Whalen CK, Steinhoff K, Wigal TL. Effects of transdermal nicotine on symptoms, moods, and cardiovascular activity in the everyday lives of smokers and nonsmokers with attention-deficit/hyperactivity disorder. *Psychology of Addictive Behavior* 2009;23:644–55.

156 Gehricke JG, Whalen CK, Jamner LD, Wigal TL, Steinhoff K. The reinforcing effects of nicotine and stimulant medication in the everyday lives of adult smokers with ADHD: A preliminary examination. *Nicotine and Tobacco Research* 2006;8:37–47.

157 Levin ED, Conners CK, Sparrow E, *et al*. Nicotine effects on adults with attention-deficit/hyperactivity disorder. *Psychopharmacology* 1996;123:55–63.

158 Gehricke JG, Loughlin SE, Whalen CK, *et al*. Smoking to self-medicate attentional and emotional dysfunctions. *Nicotine and Tobacco Research* 2007;9(suppl 4):S523–36.

159 Milberger S, Biederman J, Faraone SV, Chen L, Jones J. ADHD is associated with early initiation of cigarette smoking in children and adolescents. *Journal of the American Academy of Child and Adolescent Psychiatry* 1997;36:37–44.

160 Whalen CK, Jamner LD, Henker B, Gehricke JG, King PS. Is there a link between adolescent cigarette smoking and pharmacotherapy for ADHD? *Psychology of Addictive Behavior* 2003;17:332–5.

161 Lambert NM, Hartsough CS. Prospective study of tobacco smoking and substance dependencies among samples of ADHD and non-ADHD participants. *Journal of Learning Disabilities* 1998;31:533–44.

162 Wilens TE, Vitulano M, Upadhyaya H, *et al*. Cigarette smoking associated with attention deficit hyperactivity disorder. *Journal of Pediatrics* 2008;153:414–9.

163 Biederman J, Faraone SV, Keenan K, *et al*. Further evidence for family-genetic risk factors in attention deficit hyperactivity disorder. Patterns of comorbidity in probands and relatives psychiatrically and pediatrically referred samples. *Archives of General Psychiatry* 1992;49:728–38.

164 Coger RW, Moe KL, Serafetinides EA. Attention deficit disorder in adults and nicotine dependence: psychobiological factors in resistance to recovery? *Journal of Psychoactive Drugs* 1996;28:229–40.

165 Ott A, Slooter AJ, Hofman A, *et al*. Smoking and risk of dementia and Alzheimer's disease in a population-based cohort study: the Rotterdam Study. *The Lancet* 1998;351:1840–3.

166 Rusanen M, Rovio S, Ngandu T, *et al*. Midlife smoking, apolipoprotein E and risk of dementia and Alzheimer's disease: a population-based cardiovascular risk factors, aging and dementia study. *Dementia and Geriatric Cognitive Disorders* 2010;30:277–84.

167 Tyas SL, White LR, Petrovitch H, Webster *et al*. Mid-life smoking and late-life dementia: the Honolulu-Asia Aging Study. *Neurobiology of Aging* 2003;24:589–96.

168 Nepal B, Brown L, Ranmuthugala G. Modelling the impact of modifying lifestyle risk factors on dementia prevalence in Australian population aged 45 years and over, 2006–2051. *Australasian Journal of Ageing* 2011;29:111–16.

169 Siennicki-Lantz A, Reinprecht F, Wollmer P, Elmstahl S. Smoking-related changes in cerebral perfusion in a population of elderly men. *Neuroepidemiology* 2008;30:84–92.

170 Anstey KJ, von Sanden C, Salim A, O'Kearney R. Smoking as a risk factor for dementia and cognitive decline: a meta-analysis of prospective studies. *American Journal of Epidemiology* 2007;166:367–78.

171 Peters R, Poulter R, Warner J, *et al*. Smoking, dementia and cognitive decline in the elderly, a systematic review. *BMC Geriatrics* 2008;8:36.

172 Barnes DE, Haight TJ, Mehta KM, *et al*. Secondhand smoke, vascular disease, and dementia incidence: findings from the cardiovascular health cognition study. *American Journal of Epidemiology* 2010;171:292–302.

173 Llewellyn DJ, Lang IA, Langa KM, Naughton F, Matthews FE. Exposure to secondhand smoke and cognitive impairment in non-smokers: national cross sectional study with cotinine measurement. *British Medical Journal* 2009;338:b462.

174 Davey Smith G, Ebrahim S. What can mendelian randomisation tell us about modifiable behavioural and environmental exposures? *British Medical Journal* 2005;330:1076–9.

175 Thorgeirsson TE, Stefansson K. Genetics of smoking behavior and its consequences: the role of nicotinic acetylcholine receptors. *Biological Psychiatry* 2008;64:919–21.

176 Lewis SJ, Araya R, Smith GD, *et al*. Smoking is associated with, but does not cause, depressed mood in pregnancy – a mendelian randomization study. *PLoS One* 2011;6:e21689.

4 Epidemiology of the association between smoking and mental disorders

4.1 Introduction

It is well recognised that the prevalence of smoking, and levels of dependence on smoking, are higher among people with mental disorders. Chapter 2 provides detailed data on this association in the UK, and similar findings are reported from the USA, where the 2007 National Health Interview Survey of 23,393 non-institutionalised adults reported a prevalence of heavy smoking (≥25 cigarettes/day) of 10.3% among those without any mental disorder, 15.1% in people with bipolar disorder, 17.8% in those with schizophrenia, 19.8% in those with phobias or fears, and 28.8% in those with serious psychological distress.[1] However, as the causal nature of this association remains uncertain, it is not clear whether smoking independently increases the risk of mental disorders, or whether having a mental disorder increases the risk of becoming a smoker. A common view is that nicotine helps provide gratification and relief from anxiety and other symptoms associated with mental disorders; however, it is also possible that the symptoms of nicotine dependence are wrongly attributed to, or exacerbate symptoms of, mental disorders. This chapter reviews the literature on the association between smoking and mental disorders, and assesses whether smoking is associated with an increased risk of incidence of mental disorders, and/or whether those with mental disorders are more likely to become smokers. To do so, we have focused, where possible, on cohort or longitudinal studies in which the association between smoking and mental disorders can be assessed prospectively.

4.2 Search methods

Comprehensive searches of electronic databases (Medline, EMBASE and PsycINFO, from inception to February 2011) were carried out using search terms developed through discussion with relevant experts, to identify all cohort studies assessing: the relationship between smoking and mental health conditions, categorised into behavioural and emotion disorders (hyperkinetic disorder, conduct disorder, emotional disorder); behavioural syndromes (including eating disorders); schizophrenia, schizotypal and delusional disorders (including schizoaffective disorders and psychotic disorder); mood and affective disorders (including manic episode, bipolar affective disorder, depressive disorder); and neurotic and stress-related disorders (including anxiety disorder, obsessive–compulsive disorder, post-traumatic stress disorder). We excluded organic mental disorders (including dementia, mental and behavioural disorders due to psychoactive substance use, learning disability and disorders of psychological development). Separate literature searches were carried out to identify studies that assessed the effect of smoking on dementia and those assessing mortality and morbidity among people with mental health disorders. We also scanned and checked the reference lists from original research papers and reviewed articles to identify further eligible studies. No language restrictions were imposed during the search and translations were sought where necessary.

The systematic reviews were conducted in accordance with the Meta-analysis Of Observational Studies in Epidemiology (MOOSE) guidelines.[2] We extracted adjusted estimates of association from the publications, where available; otherwise we calculated unadjusted (crude) figures from the results presented. Where more than one method of diagnostic ascertainment of mental disorder was reported, we used estimates based on clinical diagnoses in preference to those reported by parents or teachers. Estimates of pooled relative risks (RRs) were generated, where possible, for each outcome by random effect meta-analyses using a generic inverse variance method within Review Manager software (Review Manager (RevMan), Version 5.1). Heterogeneity was quantified using I^2.

The searches identified 10,522 publications, of which 814 were selected based on the relevance of their titles. We excluded 528 of these after scrutiny of their abstracts, and screened 286 full text papers, of which 201 were excluded, largely because the association between smoking and mental disorder was not assessed prospectively. Thus, 85 studies were identified as suitable for inclusion in the following reviews, and these covered the following diagnostic groups: any mental disorder, emotional and behavioural problems, bipolar disorder, schizophrenia, anxiety, eating disorders, and depression.

4.3 Smoking and onset of any mental disorder

Three studies identified in our searches measured the onset of any mental disorder (relating to the most common mood disorders, anxiety disorders and substance use disorders) over a 12-month period among smokers and non-smokers who had no mental disorder at the start of the follow-up period.[3–5] In one of these studies, of 2,726 adults from the Netherlands, smoking was associated with a significant increase in the incidence of mental disorder in the following year (incidence rate ratio [IRR] = 1.62, 95% confidence interval [CI] 1.15–2.30),[3] but in the second, carried out in the UK and including 651 adults with learning difficulties, there was no significant effect on mental disorder incidence.[4] In the third study, smoking significantly increased the risk of psychiatric diagnoses in 6442 US Marines deployed to combat zones (hazard rate [HR] = 1.75, 95% CI 1.44–2.12).[5]

4.4 Smoking and developmental and emotional disorders

Twenty-one papers assessed the association between smoking and developmental and emotional disorders,[6–26] of which two used the same cohort of participants[14,15] (see Table A1). All of these studies assessed the effect of developmental and/or emotional disorders on the risk of becoming a smoker; only one study[16] also investigated the effect of smoking on the risk of developmental disorders. Twenty of the included studies examined the associations prospectively, and one[6] used retrospective methods. Thirteen studies were carried out in North America, five in Europe and three in Australasia. Most included data from males and females, generally in equal proportions, one study included females only[23] and three studies males only.[10,11,19]

Although all studies looked at the longitudinal relationship between developmental disorders and smoking initiation, only seven of the studies restricted their analyses to non-smokers at baseline,[7,13,15,21–24,26] but one study reported having repeated analyses excluding smokers at baseline and obtaining similar results; data were not reported, however.[12]

The range of developmental disorders assessed included attention deficit hyperactivity disorder (ADHD; seven studies[7–10,12,21,26]), conduct disorder (CD; thirteen studies[6,8–12,14,15,17,19,20,23,26]), inattention (three studies[11–13]), hyperactivity–impulsivity (three studies[11,12,15]), hyperactivity (five studies[13,14,16,19,25]), oppositional defiant disorder (three studies[11,14,26]), internalising disorder (two studies[16,22]), externalising disorder (one study[22]), and composite measures of behavioural disorders (four studies [16,18,19,24]) and emotional disorders (one study[8]).

4.4.1 Composite measures of behavioural and emotional disorders

A meta-analysis of three studies[18,19,24] demonstrated that children with behavioural disorders were at significantly increased risk of initiating smoking compared with children without behavioural disorders (RR = 1.23, 95% CI 1.07–1.42, I^2 = 0% – Fig 4.1). In addition, a meta-analysis of two studies[16,18] found that people with behavioural disorders were almost more than twice as likely to become daily/regular smokers compared with those without behavioural disorders (RR = 2.11, 95% CI 1.16–3.85, I^2 = 62% – Fig 4.1). Data from one further study found that emotional disorders were not significantly associated with smoking onset (prevalence ratio 1.13[8]).

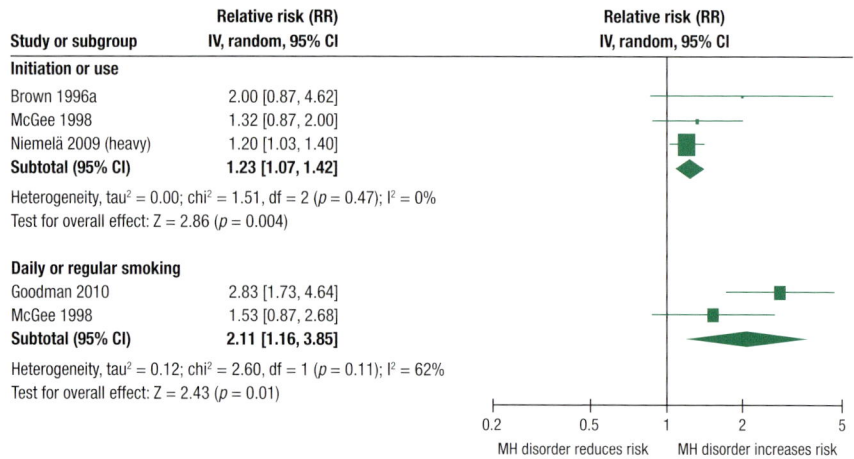

Fig 4.1 Behavioural disorders in children and adolescents and the onset of smoking. MH, mental health.

4.4.2 Internalising and externalising problems

Two studies reported the association between smoking and internalising or externalising problems.[16,22] Internalising problems were not significantly associated with smoking initiation or use (RR = 1.24, 95% CI 0.78–1.96, I^2 = 80%, two studies[16,22]), or with daily or regular smoking (RR =1.02, 95% CI 0.99–1.05, one study [22]). People with externalising problems were no more likely to initiate smoking (RR = 1.02, 95% CI 0.98–1.06), but were slightly more likely to progress to regular smoking (RR = 1.07, 95% CI 1.03–1.11), although this association is based on the findings from only one study.[22] Data from one study found that smoking was not a determinant of an increased risk of onset of internalising disorders (RR = 0.77, 95% CI 0.36–1.64).[16]

4.4.3 Attention deficit hyperactivity disorder

A meta-analysis of five studies[7,9,10,12,21] demonstrated that people with ADHD were more likely to start smoking than those without the disorder (RR = 1.75, 95% CI 1.31–2.34, I^2 = 56% – Fig 4.2). Two further studies could not be included in the meta-analysis because no suitable data were reported;[8,26] one of these reported a significant threefold increase in the risk of onset of daily smoking (RR = 3.1, p <0.001),[26] but the other reported no significant association (prevalence ratio 1.0, p >0.05).[8]

When looking at the subtypes of ADHD, pooled analyses found that hyperactivity–impulsivity was not significantly associated with smoking

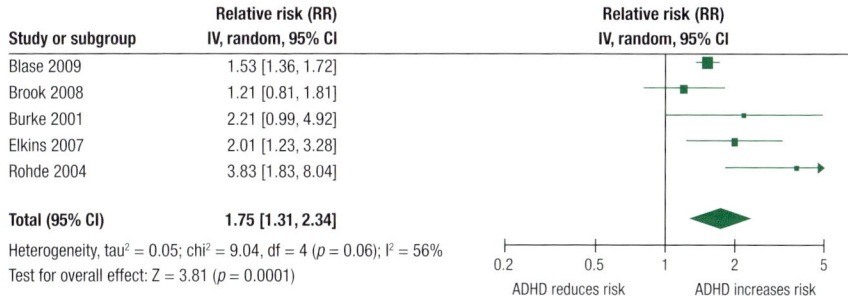

Fig 4.2 Attention deficit hyperactivity disorder (ADHD) and the onset of smoking.

initiation (RR = 1.07, 95% CI 0.91–1.26, I^2 = 71%, three studies);[11,12,15] however, smoking initiation was significantly increased in those with inattention (RR = 1.23, 95% CI 1.06–1.44, I^2 = 69%, three studies),[11–13] and particularly so in those with both inattention and hyperactivity (RR = 2.64, 95% CI 1.48–4.72).[13] There was some evidence to suggest that hyperactivity alone may be associated with smoking initiation (RR = 1.63, 95% CI 0.95–2.81, I^2 = 77%, three studies),[13,19,25] onset of daily/regular smoking (RR = 1.25, 95% CI 0.55–2.82)[16] and lifetime smoking (RR = 1.25, 95% CI 0.74–2.11),[14] but none of these results was statistically significant.

4.4.4 Oppositional defiant disorder

Three studies assessed the association between oppositional defiant disorder and smoking.[11,14,26] One found a significant twofold increase in the onset of daily smoking (RR = 2.1, p <0.007);[26] however, other studies found no significant association with smoking initiation (RR = 1.00, 95% CI 0.85–1.16),[11] lifetime smoking (RR = 1.45, 95% CI 0.72–2.91)[14] or daily smoking[14] (data not reported).

4.4.5 Conduct disorder

In a meta-analysis of five studies,[10–12,15,19] people with conduct disorder were significantly more likely to initiate smoking (RR = 1.30, 95% CI 1.17–1.44, I^2 = 18% – Fig 4.3). One of these studies also showed that children with high symptoms of both conduct disorder and hyperactivity–impulsivity were almost twice as likely to start smoking compared with children with low symptom scores for conduct disorder and hyperactivity–impulsivity (boys: HR = 1.92, 95% CI 1.03–3.59; girls: HR = 1.86, 95% CI 1.14–3.03).[15] Data from a further study that could not be included in the meta-analysis also found a significant increase in the

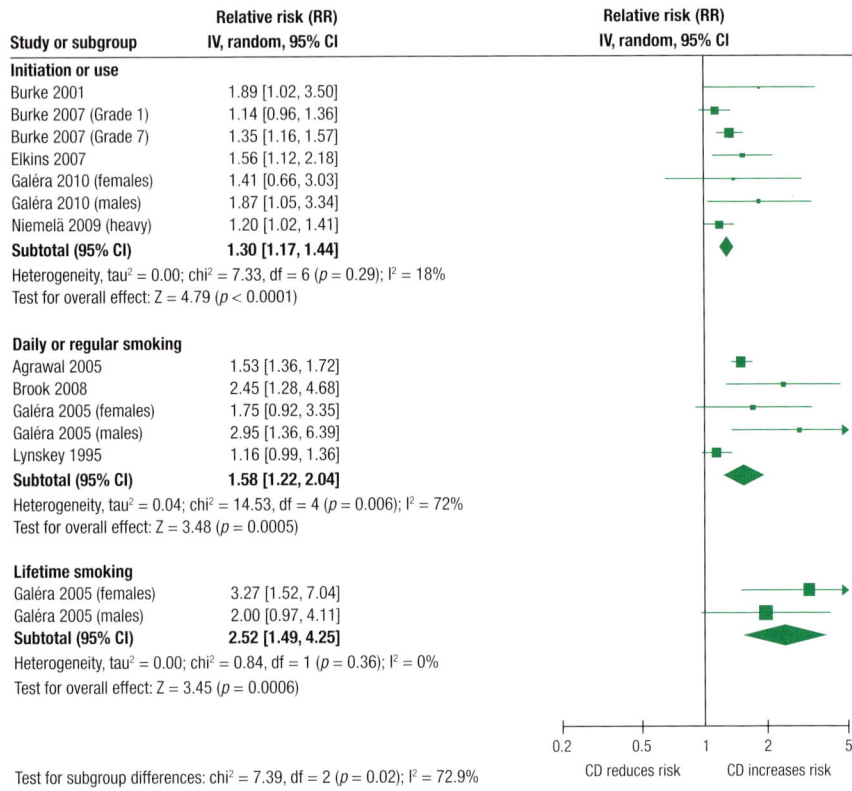

Fig 4.3 Conduct disorder (CD) and the onset of smoking.

onset of daily smoking in individuals with conduct disorder (RR = 3.8, p <0.001).[26] People with conduct disorder were also significantly more likely to become daily/regular smokers than those without the disorder (RR = 1.58, 95% CI 1.22–2.04, I^2 = 72%; four studies[6,9,14,17] – Fig 4.3), and to become lifelong smokers (RR = 2.52, 95% CI 1.49–4.25).[14] In a further three studies that could not be included in the meta-analysis, one reported a significant positive correlation between conduct disorder and tobacco use at 9 years of follow-up,[20] one reported a non-significant 61% increase in the risk of tobacco use at 4 years of follow-up[8] and in the remaining study in girls a significant 40% reduction in the onset of daily smoking was identified per unit increase in scores of behavioural conduct (where lower score reflects poorer conduct) (RR = 0.60, 95% CI 0.47–0.77).[23]

4.5 Smoking and bipolar disorder

Two longitudinal studies examined the relationship between smoking and bipolar disorder in adolescents and adults[3,27] (see Table A2). There was a non-statistically significant association between smoking and the incidence of bipolar disorder in adults (IRR = 6.45, 95% CI 0.55–75.65),[3] but numbers were small with only nine incident cases in the cohort. Conflicting results were seen for the impact of bipolar disorder on onset of smoking in adolescence, where one study showed a significant sevenfold increase in the onset of heavy smoking in adolescents (OR = 7.1, 95% CI 1.9–25.9),[27] but no significant association with onset of light/moderate smoking in adolescents (OR = 0.9, 95% CI 0.3–2.7). Furthermore, no significant association was seen between the impact of bipolar disorder on the onset of smoking in adults in two studies (OR = 0.3, 95% CI 0–3.3;[27] magnitude of effect was not reported,[3] except $p > 0.05$).

4.6 Smoking and schizophrenia

Five cohort or longitudinal studies of the association between smoking and schizophrenia were identified in our literature search, and these are summarised in Table A3. Two of these are large cohort studies of young male army recruits, from Israel and Sweden, and report conflicting results.[28,29] The study from Israel reported an almost twofold increase in the risk of incidence schizophrenia among smokers (OR = 1.94),[29] but the Swedish study, which involved a much larger sample (48,772 vs 14,248) and number of incident cases of schizophrenia (350 vs 44), found no excess risk (OR = 0.80).[28] Another study demonstrated that the time between initiation of smoking and the onset of the mental health illness was much shorter for schizophrenia than for other psychoses.[30] A more recent prospective study[31] in Danish women found that being a smoker increased the risk of developing schizophrenia spectrum disorder by about 40% (OR = 1.42, 95% CI 1.12–1.80), with some evidence that risk increased with the number of cigarettes smoked per day. The study also reported an increased risk of affective spectrum disorder in those who smoked (OR = 1.40, 95% CI 1.05–1.86). One further study recruited 48 participants aged 12–30 years with prodromal symptoms (and thus at risk of developing schizophrenia) who participated in the Cognitive Assessment and Risk Evaluation (CARE) programme.[32] The study demonstrated that nicotine use was significantly associated with the development of schizophrenia ($p = 0.005$, Fisher's exact test).[32]

Due of the lack of prospective studies, we examined an existing systematic review of schizophrenia and smoking, based on 42 cross-sectional studies from 20 countries, by de Leon and Diaz.[33] The combined OR for current smoking among those with schizophrenia, compared with the general population, was 7.2 (95% CI 6.1–8.3) and 3.3 (95% CI 3.0–3.6) among males and females, respectively, but few studies had adjusted for confounding. Combining these pooled estimates with three results reported subsequently in four published studies[34–37] produces an OR of 4.62 (95% CI 2.15–9.92, $p < 0.001$) among males, and 1.64 (95% CI 0.48–5.68, $p = 0.43$) among females. The de Leon systematic review[33] also provided the OR for current smoking among people with schizophrenia versus patients with other mental illnesses (because the characteristics between these two groups are probably more similar than between those with schizophrenia and the general population); the combined estimates were 2.3 (95% CI 2.0–2.7, 14 studies) and 1.8 (95% CI 1.5–2.3, 8 studies) for males and females, respectively.

4.7 Smoking and anxiety disorders

Table A4 summarises the main design features and findings from 18 prospective studies identified from the literature search. Due to the different methods of assessments and definitions of exposures and outcome measures, a formal meta-analysis was not performed.

Eleven studies investigated whether people with anxiety disorders were more likely either to be smokers or to take up smoking.[21,23,24,38–45] Of these, five reported clear positive associations,[23,38–41] five found non-significant positive correlations[21,24,42–44] and one[45] found a decreased risk. Of studies of the uptake of smoking in relation to anxiety at baseline,[21,24,39–41] two found strong increases in risk (OR = 3.85, 95% CI 1.34–11.0[39] and OR = 1.9, 95% CI 1.3–2.8[41]) whereas three found modest or non-significant associations.[21,24,40]

Eight studies examined whether smokers at baseline were more likely to develop anxiety disorders later.[3,26,43,46–50] Five of these were based on teenagers and three on adults (18–64 years). ORs for onset of anxiety were increased in six of the studies that reported effect sizes: 5.53 (95% CI 1.84–16.66),[50] 1.88 (95% CI 1.15–3.06),[3] 1.46 (95% CI 1.15–1.86),[49] 3.23 (95% CI 1.0–10.8)[46] and 2.32 (95% CI 1.19–4.53).[47] Increased risks were also seen in the two studies of effect of smoking on post-traumatic stress disorder: 5.1 (95% CI 1.2–21.5)[48] and 2.64 (95% CI 1.05–6.62).[47] One study reported a positive regression coefficient between baseline smoking status and subsequent anxiety score.[43] Only one study reported a reduced risk associated with daily smoking; however, this effect was not statistically significant (RR = 0.9, $p = 0.8$).[26]

4.8 Smoking and eating disorders

Three prospective cohort studies of the association between eating disorders and the onset of smoking were identified[51–53] (see Table A5), all involving 1 year of follow-up in adolescents aged 11–15 years at baseline. In one of the studies, binge eating or purging was not significantly related to smoking uptake in males (OR = 0.7, 95% CI 0.1–4.1) or females (binge eating: OR = 1.8, 95% CI 0.9–3.5; purging: OR = 2.0, 95% CI 0.8–4.9).[51] However, in the other two studies, the risk of onset of smoking was found to be significantly associated with body dissatisfaction and/or eating pathology (OR = 4.33, 95% CI 1.71–10.95),[52] and in those with a high eating disorder symptom score in girls (OR = 2.15, 95% CI 1.16–3.97) but not in boys (OR = 1.67, 95% CI 0.91–3.07).[53] One of the included studies also assessed the relationship between smoking and onset of eating disorders,[51] and found no clear association between smoking and the incidence of purging (OR = 0.9, 95% CI 0.3–2.5) or binge eating (OR = 1.4, 95% CI 0.6–3.0) in females.[51]

4.9 Smoking and depression

We identified 47 longitudinal studies of smoking and depression in our searches.[3,21,24,26,27,47,54–94] One cohort was reported in two studies,[63,84] the Add Health cohort in three studies,[55,80,93] and the Teenage Attitudes and Practices Survey (TAPS) also in three studies[54,78,83] (see Table A6).

4.9.1 Smoking and onset of depression

There were 32 studies of the effect of smoking on the onset of depression, most of which included males and females combined and some of which provided gender-specific estimates for males[54–58,60] or females;[54–56,59,60,76,90,91] the latter group included three studies of postpartum depression.[76,90,91]

A meta-analysis of 26 studies found regular or daily smoking significantly increased the risk of onset of depression by 52% (RR = 1.52, 95% CI 1.36–1.71; $I^2 = 68\%$ – Fig 4.4),[24,47,54–75,86,87] with a slightly larger magnitude of effect in females (RR = 1.79, 95% CI 1.24–2.58) than in males (RR = 1.39, 95% CI 1.15–1.68). Similar findings were seen in two studies that could not be included in the meta-analysis (IRR = 1.28, 95% CI 0.76–2.16;[3] light smoking: HR = 1.29, 95% CI 0.74–2.25; moderate smoking: HR = 2.01, 95% CI 1.17–3.43; heavy smoking: HR = 4.34, 95% CI 1.85–10.18[94]); however, no effect was seen in a further study assessing the association between daily smoking and the onset of a depressive disorder (RR = 1.0, $p = 0.9$[26]). A subgroup analysis of the 26 studies found similar magnitudes of effect for the association between smoking and the onset of depression in adolescents (RR = 1.49, 95% CI 1.25–1.77, $I^2 = 69\%$, 11 studies) and in adults (RR = 1.56, 95% CI 1.32–1.83, $I^2 = 67\%$, 15 studies) (test for subgroup difference $p = 0.71$) (Fig 4.5).

A meta-analysis of six studies found that ex-smokers were no more likely to develop depression than never smokers (RR = 1.02, 95% CI 0.82–1.27, $I^2 = 60\%$),[56–58,60,71,75] and one study found no significant association between being a former smoker and the risk of onset of depression compared with being a current smoker (RR = 0.88, 95% CI 0.56–1.40).[86]

Three studies[76,90,91] (see Table A6) assessed the association between smoking and postpartum depression and revealed a twofold increase in the risk of development of postpartum depression in women who were smokers during pregnancy (RR = 2.08, 95% CI 1.50–2.91, $I^2 = 0\%$ – Fig 4.6).

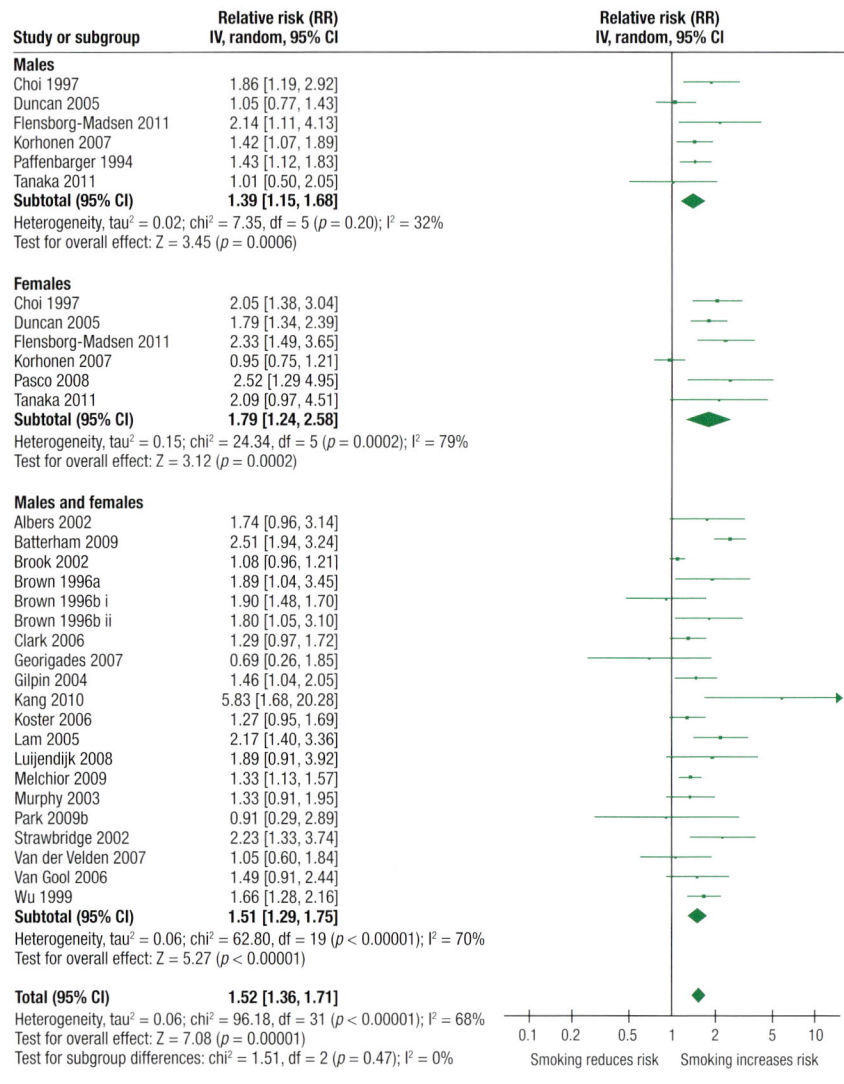

Fig 4.4 Smoking behaviour on onset of depression.

4.9.2 Depression and onset of smoking

A meta-analysis of 10 studies found that depression was significantly associated with the onset of smoking by 43% (RR = 1.43, 95% CI 1.17–1.74, I^2 = 71% – Fig 4.7).[24,27,70,77,79–83,87] One cohort of individuals, included in the meta-analysis, also reported a 30% significant increase in smoking initiation in those with a high baseline depressive symptom score (OR = 1.3, 95% CI 1.1–1.6).[78] One further study, which could not be included in the meta-analysis, found no significant association between high depressive symptoms and onset of smoking in

Epidemiology of the association between smoking and mental disorders 4

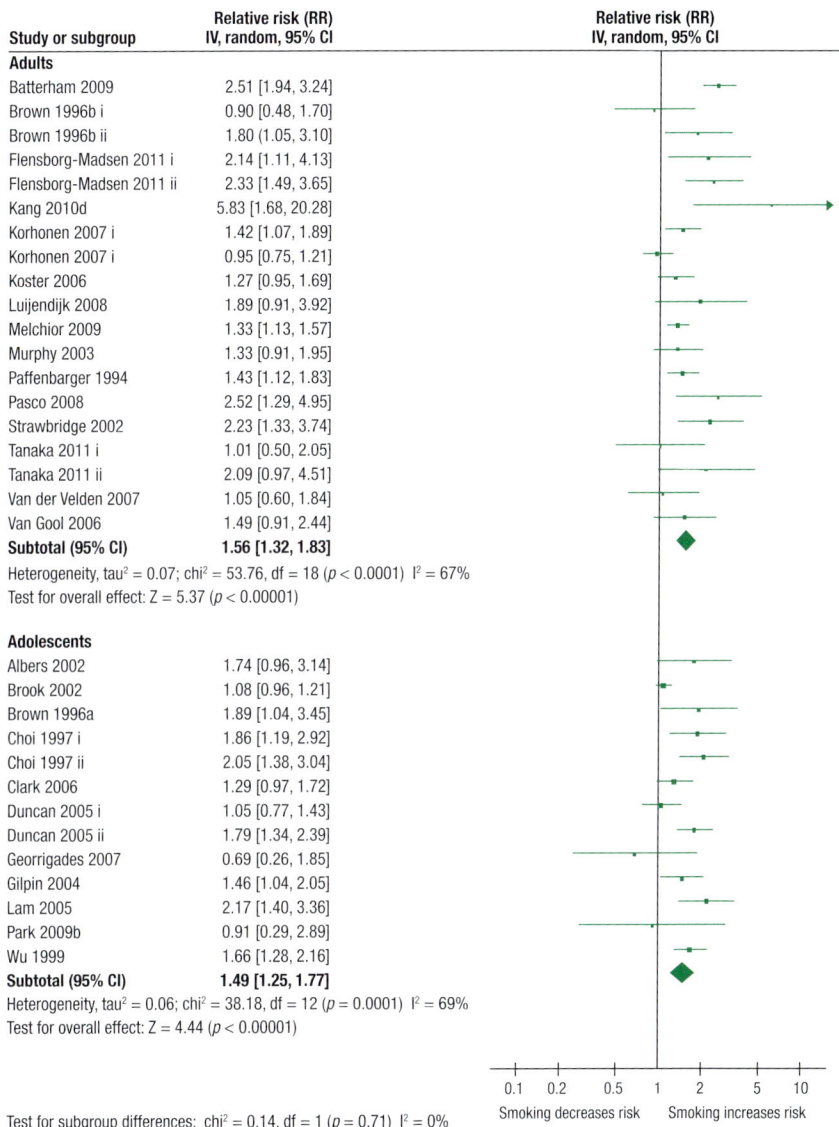

Fig 4.5 Smoking and the onset of depression: subgroup analysis based on age of population.

adolescent girls; however, the study reported a modest significant increase in the onset of smoking with high depressive symptoms in boys (HR = 1.03, p <0.01).[92]

A meta-analysis of 10 studies found that depression was significantly associated with a 34% increased risk of the onset of daily/regular smoking (RR = 1.34, 95% CI 1.13–1.58, I^2 = 80% – Fig 4.8).[21,68,74,77,81,83–85,88,89] However, one study, which could not be included in the meta-analysis, found no significant association

Smoking and mental health

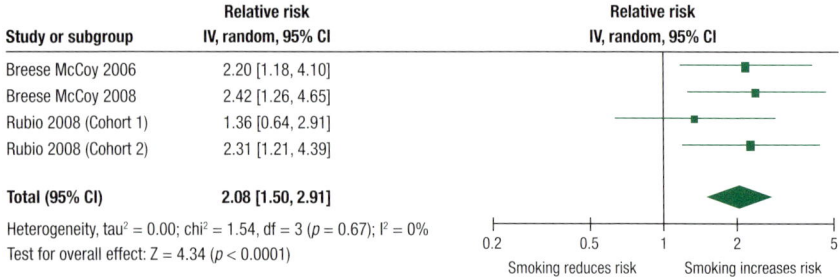

Fig 4.6 Smoking and onset of postpartum depression.

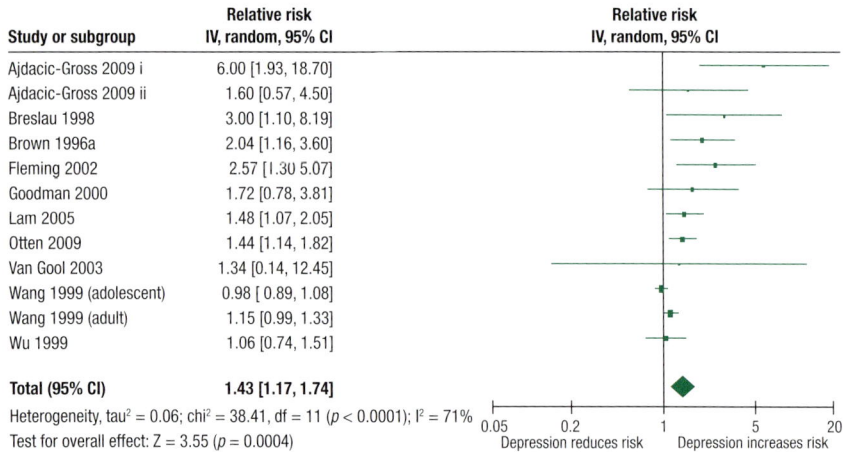

Fig 4.7 Depression and the onset of smoking.

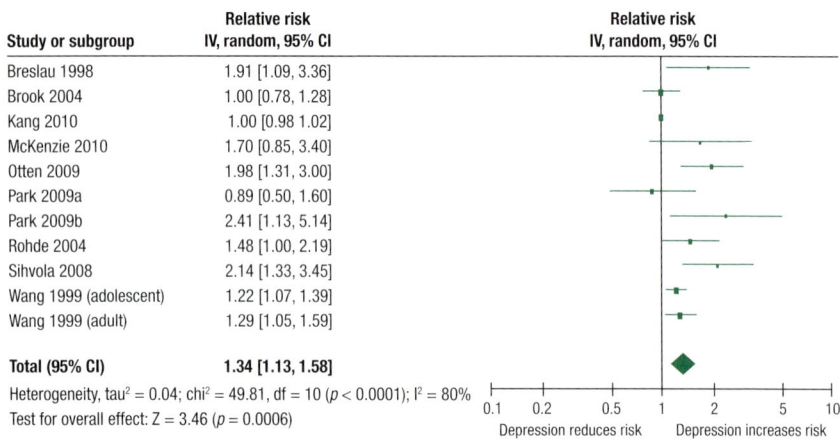

Fig 4.8 Depression and the risk of daily/regular smoking.

between per unit increase in depression score at baseline and the transition to daily smoking 1 year later (OR = 1.01, 95% CI 0.99–1.02).[93]

4.10 Smoking and dementia

In 2007, Anstey *et al* reported a review and meta-analysis of 19 studies published before June 2005 with at least 12 months of follow-up, including data from over 26,000 participants followed from 2 years to 30 years with respect to incident dementia and/or cognitive decline.[95] The pooled relative risk for developing dementia was estimated as 1.27 (95% CI 1.02–1.60, two studies) in current smokers compared with never smokers, and corresponding relative risks of incident Alzheimer's disease and vascular dementia were 1.79 (95% CI 1.43–2.23, four studies) and 1.78 (95% CI 1.28–2.47, two studies), respectively. A second systematic review and meta-analysis published in 2008 was conducted in parallel with the first review, but included more contemporary studies written in English language and published up to November 2007.[96] The second review reported essentially similar findings, with a pooled ratio for current smoking and incident Alzheimer's disease of 1.59 (95% CI 1.15–2.20, eight studies). The four larger studies found positive associations between current smoking and incident dementia (or subtypes), and include a 4-year follow-up of 1,064 participants aged 65 years and over,[97] a 2-year follow-up of 2,820 participants aged 60 years and over,[98] a follow-up of 6,870 people aged at least 55 years over an average period of 2.1 years,[99] and an association between mid-life smoking and late-life Alzheimer's disease in 3,734 men with a mean age of around 77 years.[100] Of these, two reported exposure-related effects, where the risk of dementia increased with increasing cigarette consumption.[98,100]

However, the large studies that found no association between smoking and an increased risk of dementia include the Canadian Study of Health and Aging (RR = 0.82, 95% CI 0.57–1.17)[101] and the MRC Cognitive Function and Ageing Study (RR = 0.90, 95% CI 0.50–1.50).[102] The reason for this heterogeneity is unclear, although both studies involved relatively long follow-up periods and findings from the Rotterdam cohort study have suggested a diminution of risk ratio for all dementia from 2.2 at approximately 2 years[99] to 1.5 at approximately 7 years;[103] it is therefore possible that longer follow-up periods in panel survey designs obscure the effect because of selective attrition. Relevant studies published since the systematic reviews mentioned above include two that report positive associations between smoking and dementia hospitalisation or healthcare contacts,[104,105] and one reporting a strong association between mid-life smoking status and late-life dementia risk in 1449 people aged 65–79 years.[106] A recent review also concluded that studies with tobacco industry affiliation were more likely to report a protective effect and less likely to report a risk effect than studies without such affiliation.[107]

4.11 Smoking and increased mortality and morbidity among people with mental disorders

It is plausible that people with mental disorders might have higher rates of mortality or major morbidity because of their mental disorders, or their high prevalence of smoking. The excess risk of death or morbidity among those with mental health disorders has been studied in several reports, and Table A7 summarises the main findings from large prospective studies (>20,000 participants).[108–124] People with mental health problems, such as depression and schizophrenia, appear to have a higher risk of cardiovascular disease and stroke, even after adjustment for smoking status (never, former and current). There may be some excess risk of cardiovascular death due to antipsychotic medications.[125] There was no consistent evidence for an increased risk for cancer among people with mental disorders, which is surprising given that smoking has substantial significant effects on several common cancers. One study of a cohort of 4,825 American patients[126] compared age-adjusted death rates (with allowance for other confounding factors) in people with or without mental disorders in relation to smoking status. The hazard ratio for cancer among current smokers was 2.80 (95% CI 0.65–11.94) and 1.96 (95% CI 1.16–3.34) for those with and without chronically depressed mood respectively (the reference group was non-smokers without depressed mood).

4.12 Summary

> - Current smoking is associated with an increased risk of onset of depression, including postnatal depression, and people with depression are more likely to become smokers.
> - Current smoking is associated with an increased risk of onset of anxiety disorders, and people with anxiety disorders are more likely to take up smoking.
> - Former smokers are not at an increased risk of subsequent onset of depression.
> - Adolescents with eating disorders are more likely to become smokers.
> - There is some evidence that people with behavioural disorders, particularly ADHD and conduct disorder, are more likely to become smokers, but no evidence that smoking increases the risk of onset of these conditions.
> - There is a strong association between smoking and schizophrenia in cross-sectional studies, but longitudinal evidence on the temporal relationship is mixed.
> - Adolescents with bipolar disorder may be more likely to become heavy smokers.
> - Smoking is associated with an increased risk of dementia.
> - People with mental disorders appear to have higher risks of cardiovascular disease and stroke (after accounting for the effects of smoking); however, there is no consistent evidence regarding an increased risk of cancer.

The appendix to Chapter 4 (Tables A1–7) is available online at
www.rcplondon.ac.uk/publications/smoking-and-mental-health.

References

1 McClave AK, McKnight-Eily LR, Davis SP, Dube SR. Smoking characteristics of adults with selected lifetime mental illnesses: results from the 2007 National Health Interview Survey. *American Journal of Public Health* 2010;100:2464–72.

2 Stroup DF, Berlin JA, Morton SC, *et al*. Meta-analysis of observational studies in epidemiology: a proposal for reporting. Meta-analysis Of Observational Studies in Epidemiology (MOOSE) group. *Journal of the American Medical Association* 2000;283:2008–12.

3 Cuijpers P, Smit F, ten Have M, de Graaf R. Smoking is associated with first-ever incidence of mental disorders: a prospective population-based study. *Addiction* 2007;102:1303–9.

4 Smiley E, Cooper SA, Finlayson J, *et al*. Incidence and predictors of mental ill-health in adults with intellectual disabilities: prospective study. *British Journal of Psychiatry* 2007;191:313–19.

5 Larson GE, Booth-Kewley S, Highfill-McRoy RM, Young SYN. Prospective analysis of psychiatric risk factors in marines sent to war. *Military Medicine* 2009;174:737–44.

6 Agrawal A, Madden PAF, Heath AC, *et al*. Correlates of regular cigarette smoking in a population-based sample of Australian twins. *Addiction* 2005;100:1709–19.

7 Blase SL, Gilbert AN, Anastopoulos AD, *et al*. Self-reported ADHD and adjustment in college: Cross-sectional and longitudinal findings. *Journal of Attention Disorders* 2009;13:297–309.

8 Boyle MH, Offord DR, Racine YA, *et al*. Predicting substance use in early adolescence based on parent and teacher assessments of childhood psychiatric disorder: results from the Ontario Child Health Study follow-up. *Journal of Child Psychology and Psychiatry, and Allied Disciplines* 1993;34:535–44.

9 Brook JS, Duan T, Zhang C, Cohen PR, Brook DW. The association between attention deficit hyperactivity disorder in adolescence and smoking in adulthood. *American Journal on Addictions* 2008;17:54–9.

10 Burke JD, Loeber R, Lahey BB. Which aspects of ADHD are associated with tobacco use in early adolescence? *Journal of Child Psychology and Psychiatry and Allied Disciplines* 2001;42:493–502.

11 Burke JD, Loeber R, White HR, Stouthamer-Loeber M, Pardini DA. Inattention as a key predictor of tobacco use in adolescence. *Journal of Abnormal Psychology* 2007;116:249–59.

12 Elkins IJ, McGue M, Iacono WG. Prospective effects of attention-deficit/hyperactivity disorder, conduct disorder, and sex on adolescent substance use and abuse. *Archives of General Psychiatry* 2007;64:1145–52.

13 Fuemmeler BF, Kollins SH, McClernon FJ. Attention deficit hyperactivity disorder symptoms predict nicotine dependence and progression to regular smoking from adolescence to young adulthood. *Journal of Pediatric Psychology* 2007;32:1203–13.

14 Galéra C, Fombonne E, Chastang JF, Bouvard M. Childhood hyperactivity-inattention symptoms and smoking in adolescence. *Drug and Alcohol Dependence* 2005;78:101–8.

15 Galéra C, Bouvard M, Melchior M, *et al*. Disruptive symptoms in childhood and adolescence and early initiation of tobacco and cannabis use: The Gazel Youth study. *European Psychiatry* 2010;25:402–8.

16 Goodman A. Substance use and common child mental health problems: examining longitudinal associations in a British sample. *Addiction* 2010;105:1484–96.

17 Lynskey MT, Fergusson DM. Childhood conduct problems, attention deficit behaviors, and adolescent alcohol, tobacco, and illicit drug use. *Journal of Abnormal Child Psychology* 1995;23:281–302.

18 McGee, R, Williams S, Stanton W. Is mental health in childhood a major predictor of smoking in adolescence? *Addiction* 1998;93:1869–74.

19 Niemelä S, Sourander A, Pilowsky DJ, et al. Childhood antecedents of being a cigarette smoker in early adulthood. The Finnish 'From a Boy to a Man' Study. *Journal of Child Psychology and Psychiatry and Allied Disciplines* 2009;50:343–51.

20 Pine DS, Cohen P, Brook J, Coplan JD. Psychiatric symptoms in adolescence as predictors of obesity in early adulthood: a longitudinal study. *American Journal of Public Health* 1997;87:1303–10.

21 Rohde P, Kahler CW, Lewinsohn PM, Brown RA. Psychiatric disorders, familial factors, and cigarette smoking: II. Associations with progression to daily smoking. *Nicotine and Tobacco Research* 2004;6:119–32.

22 Spein AR, Sexton H, Kvernmo S. Predictors of smoking behaviour among indigenous Sami adolescents and non-indigenous peers in North Norway. *Scandinavian Journal of Public Health* 2004;32:118–29.

23 Voorhees CC, Schreiber GB, Schumann BC, Biro F, Crawford PB. Early predictors of daily smoking in young women: the national heart, lung, and blood institute growth and health study. *Preventive Medicine* 2002;34:616–24.

24 Brown RA, Lewinsohn PM, Seeley JR, Wagner EF. Cigarette smoking, major depression, and other psychiatric disorders among adolescents. *Journal of the American Academy of Child and Adolescent Psychiatry* 1996;35:1602–10.

25 Barkley RA, Fischer M, Edelbrock CS, Smallish L. The adolescent outcome of hyperactive children diagnosed by research criteria: I. An 8-year prospective follow-up study. *Journal of the American Academy of Child and Adolescent Psychiatry* 1990;29:546–57.

26 Clark DB, Cornelius J. Childhood psychopathology and adolescent cigarette smoking: A prospective survival analysis in children at high risk for substance use disorders. *Addictive Behaviors* 2004;29:837–841.

27 Ajdacic-Gross V, Landolt K, Angst J, et al. Adult versus adolescent onset of smoking: How are mood disorders and other risk factors involved? *Addiction* 2009;104:1411–19.

28 Zammit S, Allebeck P, Dalman C, et al. Investigating the association between cigarette smoking and schizophrenia in a cohort study. *American Journal of Psychiatry* 2003;160:2216–21.

29 Weiser, M, Reichenberg A, Grotto I, et al. Higher rates of cigarette smoking in male adolescents before the onset of schizophrenia: A historical-prospective cohort study. *American Journal of Psychiatry* 2004;161:1219–23.

30 Riala K, Hakko H, Isohanni M, Pouta A, Rasanen P. Is initiation of smoking associated with the prodromal phase of schizophrenia? *Journal of Psychiatry and Neuroscience* 2005;30:26–32.

31 Sorensen HJ, Mortensen EL, Reinisch JM, Mednick SA. A prospective study of smoking in young women and risk of later psychiatric hospitalization. *Nordic Journal of Psychiatry* 2011;65:3–8.

32 Kristensen K, Cadenhead KS. Cannabis abuse and risk of psychosis in a prodromal sample. *Psychiatry Research* 2007;151:151–4.

33 de Leon J, Diaz FJ. A meta-analysis of worldwide studies demonstrates an association between schizophrenia and tobacco smoking behaviors. *Schizophrenia Research* 2005;76:135–57.

34 Subramaniam M, Cheok C, Lee IM, et al. Nicotine dependence and psychiatric disorders among young males in Singapore. *Nicotine and Tobacco Research* 2009;11:1107–13.

35 Zhang XY, Li CB, Li M, *et al.* Smoking initiation and schizophrenia: a replication study in a Chinese Han population. *Schizophrenia Research* 2010;119:110–14.

36 Zhang XY, Zhang RL, Pan M, *et al.* Sex difference in the prevalence of smoking in Chinese schizophrenia. *Journal of Psychiatric Research* 2010;44:986–8.

37 Campo-Arias, A, Díaz-Martínez LA, Rueda-Jaimes GE, *et al.* Smoking is associated with schizophrenia, but not with mood disorders, within a population with low smoking rates: a matched case-control study in Bucaramanga, Colombia. *Schizophrenia Research* 2006;83:269–276.

38 Patton GC, Carlin JB, Coffey C, *et al.* Depression, anxiety, and smoking initiation: a prospective study over 3 years. *American Journal of Public Health* 1998;88:1518–22.

39 Sonntag H, Wittchen HU, Hofler M, Kessler RC, Stein MB. Are social fears and DSM-IV social anxiety disorder associated with smoking and nicotine dependence in adolescents and young adults? *European Psychiatry: the Journal of the Association of European Psychiatrists* 2000;15:67–74.

40 Marmorstein NR, White HR, Loeber R, Stouthamer-Loeber M. Anxiety as a predictor of age at first use of substances and progression to substance use problems among boys. *Journal of Abnormal Child Psychology* 2010;38:211–24.

41 Swendsen J, Conway KP, Degenhardt L, *et al.* Mental disorders as risk factors for substance use, abuse and dependence: Results from the 10-year follow-up of the National Comorbidity Survey. *Addiction* 2010;105:1117–1128.

42 Ferdinand RF, Blum, M Verhulst FC. Psychopathology in adolescence predicts substance use in young adulthood. *Addiction* 2001;96:861–70.

43 Pedersen W, von Soest T. Smoking, nicotine dependence and mental health among young adults: A 13-year population-based longitudinal study. *Addiction* 2009;104:129–37.

44 Woodward LJ, Fergusson DM. Life course outcomes of young people with anxiety disorders in adolescence. *Journal of the American Academy of Child and Adolescent Psychiatry* 2001;40:1086–93.

45 Johnson EO, Novak SP. Onset and persistence of daily smoking: The interplay of socioeconomic status, gender, and psychiatric disorders. *Drug and Alcohol Dependence* 2009;104(suppl 1):S50–7.

46 Patel V, Kirkwood BR, Pednekar S, Weiss H, Mabey D. Risk factors for common mental disorders in women. *British Journal of Psychiatry* 2006;189:547–55.

47 Van der Velden PG, Grievink L, Olff M, Gersons BPR, Kleber RJ. Smoking as a risk factor for mental health disturbances after a disaster: a prospective comparative study. *Journal of Clinical Psychiatry* 2007;68:87–92.

48 Isensee B, Wittchen H-U, Stein MB, Hofler M, Lieb R. Smoking increases the risk of panic: findings from a prospective community study. *Archives of General Psychiatry* 2003;60:692–700.

49 John U, Meyer C, Rumpf HJ, Hapke U. Smoking, nicotine dependence and psychiatric comorbidity – A population-based study including smoking cessation after three years. *Drug and Alcohol Dependence* 2004;76:287–95.

50 Johnson JG, Cohen P, Pine DS, *et al.* Association between cigarette smoking and anxiety disorders during adolescence and early adulthood. *Journal of the American Medical Association* 2000;284:2348–51.

51 Field AE, Austin SB, Frazier AL, *et al.* Smoking, getting drunk, and engaging in bulimic behaviors: in which order are the behaviors adopted? *Journal of the American Academy of Child and Adolescent Psychiatry* 2002;41:846–53.

52 Stice E, Shaw H. Prospective relations of body image, eating, and affective disturbances to smoking onset in adolescent girls: how Virginia slims. *Journal of Consulting and Clinical Psychology* 2003;71:129–35.

53 French SA, Perry CL, Leon GR, Fulkerson JA. Weight concerns, dieting behavior, and smoking initiation among adolescents: a prospective study. *American Journal of Public Health* 1994;84:1818–20.

54 Choi WS, Patten CA, Gillin JC, Kaplan RM, Pierce JP. Cigarette smoking predicts development of depressive symptoms among U.S. adolescents. *Annals of Behavioral Medicine* 1997;19:42–50.

55 Duncan B, Rees DI. Effect of smoking on depressive symptomatology: A reexamination of data from the National Longitudinal Study of Adolescent Health. *American Journal of Epidemiology* 2005;162:461–70.

56 Flensborg-Madsen Trine T, Bay von Scholten M, Flachs EM, *et al.* Tobacco smoking as a risk factor for depression. A 26-year population-based follow-up study. *Journal of Psychiatric Research* 2011;45:143–9.

57 Korhonen T, B Ulla, Varjonen J, *et al.* Smoking behaviour as a predictor of depression among Finnish men and women: A prospective cohort study of adult twins. *Psychological Medicine* 2007;37:705–15.

58 Paffenbarger RS Jr, Lee IM, Leung R. Physical activity and personal characteristics associated with depression and suicide in American college men. *Acta Psychiatrica Scandinavica Supplementum* 1994;377:16–22.

59 Pasco JA, Williams LJ, Jacka FN, *et al.* Tobacco smoking as a risk factor for major depressive disorder: population-based study. *British Journal of Psychiatry* 2008;193:322–6.

60 Tanaka H, Sasazawa Y, Suzuki S, Nakazawa M, Koyama H. Health status and lifestyle factors as predictors of depression in middle-aged and elderly Japanese adults: A seven-year follow-up of the Komo-Ise cohort study. *BMC Psychiatry* 2011;11:20.

61 Albers AB, Biener L. The role of smoking and rebelliousness in the development of depressive symptoms among a cohort of Massachusetts adolescents. *Preventive Medicine* 2002;34:625–31.

62 Batterham PJ, Christensen H, Mackinnon AJ. Modifiable risk factors predicting major depressive disorder at four year follow-up: A decision tree approach. *BMC Psychiatry* 2009;9:75–82.

63 Brook DW, Brook JS, Zhang C, Cohen P, Whiteman M. Drug use and the risk of major depressive disorder, alcohol dependence, and substance use disorders. *Archives of General Psychiatry* 2002;59:1039–44.

64 Brown DR, Croft JB, Anda RF, Barrett DH. Evaluation of smoking on the physical activity and depressive symptoms relationship. *Medicine and Science in Sports and Exercise* 1996;28:233–40.

65 Clark C, Haines MM, Head J, *et al.* Psychological symptoms and physical health and health behaviours in adolescents: A prospective 2-year study in East London. *Addiction* 2006;102:126–35.

66 Georgiades K, Boyle MH. Adolescent tobacco and cannabis use: Young adult outcomes from the Ontario Child Health Study. *Journal of Child Psychology and Psychiatry and Allied Disciplines* 2007;48:724–31.

67 Gilpin EA, Lee L, Pierce JP. Does adolescent perception of difficulty in getting cigarettes deter experimentation? *Preventive Medicine* 2004;38:485–91.

68 Kang E, Lee J. A longitudinal study on the causal association between smoking and depression. *Journal of Preventive Medicine and Public Health* 2010;43:193–204.

69 Koster A, Bosma H, Kempen GIJM, *et al.* Socioeconomic differences in incident depression in older adults: The role of psychosocial factors, physical health status, and behavioral factors. *Journal of Psychosomatic Research* 2006;61:619–27.

70 Lam TH, Stewart SM, Ho SY, *et al.* Depressive symptoms and smoking among Hong Kong Chinese adolescents. *Addiction* 2005;100:1003–11.

71 Luijendijk HJ, Stricker BH, Hofman A, Witteman JCM, Tiemeier H. Cerebrovascular risk factors and incident depression in community-dwelling elderly. *Acta Psychiatrica Scandinavica* 2008;118:139–48.

72 Melchior M, Ferrie JE, Alexanderson K, et al. Using sickness absence records to predict future depression in a working population: Prospective findings from the GAZEL cohort. *American Journal of Public Health* 2009;99:1417–22.

73 Murphy JM, Horton NJ, Monson RR, et al. Cigarette smoking in relation to depression: historical trends from the Stirling County Study. *American Journal of Psychiatry* 2003;160:1663–9.

74 Park S. The causal association between smoking and depression among South Korean adolescents. *Journal of Addictions Nursing* 2009;20:93–103.

75 Strawbridge WJ, Deleger S, Roberts RE, Kaplan GA. Physical activity reduces the risk of subsequent depression for older adults. *American Journal of Epidemiology* 2002;156:328–34.

76 Rubio DM, Kraemer KL, Farrell MH, Day NL. Factors associated with alcohol use, depression, and their co-occurrence during pregnancy. *Alcoholism: Clinical and Experimental Research* 2008;32:1543–51.

77 Breslau, N, Peterson EL, Schultz LR, Chilcoat HD, Andreski P. Major depression and stages of smoking: A longitudinal investigation. *Archives of General Psychiatry* 1998;55:161–6.

78 Escobedo LG, Reddy M, Giovino GA. The relationship between depressive symptoms and cigarette smoking in US adolescents. *Addiction* 1998;93:433–40.

79 Fleming CB, Kim H, Harachi TW, Catalano RF. Family processes for children in early elementary school as predictors of smoking initiation. *Journal of Adolescent Health* 2002;30:184–9.

80 Goodman E, Capitman J. Depressive symptoms and cigarette smoking among teens. *Pediatrics* 2000;106:748–55.

81 Otten R, Van de Ven MOM, Engels RCME, Van den Eijnden RJJM. Depressive mood and smoking onset: A comparison of adolescents with and without asthma. *Psychology and Health* 2009;24:287–300.

82 van Gool CH, Kempen GIJM, Penninx BWJH, et al. Relationship between changes in depressive symptoms and unhealthy lifestyles in late middle aged and older persons: results from the Longitudinal Aging Study Amsterdam. *Age and Ageing* 2003;32:81–7.

83 Wang MQ, Fitzhugh EC, Green BL, et al. Prospective social-psychological factors of adolescent smoking progression. *Journal of Adolescent Health* 1999;24:2–9.

84 Brook JS, Schuster E, Zhang C. Cigarette smoking and depressive symptoms: a longitudinal study of adolescents and young adults. *Psychological Reports* 2004;95:159–66.

85 McKenzie M, Olsson CA, Jorm AF, Romaniuk H, Patton GC. Association of adolescent symptoms of depression and anxiety with daily smoking and nicotine dependence in young adulthood: findings from a 10-year longitudinal study. *Addiction* 2010;105:1652–9.

86 van Gool CH, Kempen GI, Bosma H, et al. Associations between lifestyle and depressed mood: Longitudinal results from the Maastricht Aging Study. *American Journal of Public Health* 2006;97:887–94.

87 Wu LT, Anthony JC. Tobacco smoking and depressed mood in late childhood and early adolescence. *American Journal of Public Health* 1999;89:1837–40.

88 Park ER, Chang Y, Quinn V, et al. The association of depressive, anxiety, and stress symptoms and postpartum relapse to smoking: a longitudinal study. *Nicotine and Tobacco Research* 2009;11:707–14.

89 Sihvola E, Rose RJ, Dick DM, et al. Early-onset depressive disorders predict the use of addictive substances in adolescence: a prospective study of adolescent Finnish twins. *Addiction* 2008;103:2045–53.

90 McCoy SJB, Beal JM, Saunders B, *et al*. Risk factors for postpartum depression: a retrospective investigation. *Journal of Reproductive Medicine* 2008;53:166–70.

91 Beese McCoy SJ, Beal JM, Shipman SBM, Payton ME, Watson GH. Risk factors for postpartum depression: a retrospective investigation at 4-weeks postnatal and a review of the literature. *Journal of the American Osteopathic Association* 2006;106:193–8.

92 Killen JD, Robinson TN, Haydel KF, *et al*. Prospective study of risk factors for the initiation of cigarette smoking. *Journal of Consulting and Clinical Psychology* 1997;65:1011–16.

93 Kandel DB, Kiros G-E, Schaffran C, Hu M-C. Racial/ethnic differences in cigarette smoking initiation and progression to daily smoking: a multilevel analysis. *American Journal of Public Health* 2004;94:128–35.

94 Klungsoyr O, Nygard JF, Sorensen T, Sandanger I. Cigarette smoking and incidence of first depressive episode: An 11-year, population-based follow-up study. *American Journal of Epidemiology* 2006;163:421–32.

95 Anstey KJ, von Sanden C, Salim A, O'Kearney R. Smoking as a risk factor for dementia and cognitive decline: a meta-analysis of prospective studies. *Am J Epidemiol* 2007;166:367–78.

96 Peters R, Poulter R, Warner J, *et al*. Smoking, dementia and cognitive decline in the elderly, a systematic review. *BMC Geriatrics* 2008;8:36.

97 Aggarwal NT, Bienias JL, Bennett DA, *et al*. The relation of cigarette smoking to incident Alzheimer's disease in a biracial urban community population. *Neuroepidemiology* 2006;26:140–6.

98 Juan D, Zhou DH, Li J, *et al*. A 2-year follow-up study of cigarette smoking and risk of dementia. *European Journal of Neurology* 2004;11:277–82.

99 Ott A, Slooter AJ, Hofman A, *et al*. Smoking and risk of dementia and Alzheimer's disease in a population-based cohort study: the Rotterdam Study. *The Lancet* 1998;351:1840–3.

100 Tyas SL, White LR, Petrovitch H, *et al*. Mid-life smoking and late-life dementia: the Honolulu-Asia Aging Study. *Neurobiological Aging* 2003;24:589–96.

101 Lindsay J, Laurin D, Verreault R, *et al*. Risk factors for Alzheimer's disease: a prospective analysis from the Canadian Study of Health and Aging. *American Journal of Epidemiology* 2002;156:445–53.

102 Yip AG, Brayne C, Matthews FE. Risk factors for incident dementia in England and Wales: The Medical Research Council Cognitive Function and Ageing Study. A population-based nested case-control study. *Age and Ageing* 2006;35:154–60.

103 Reitz C, den Heijer T, van Duijn C, Hofman A, Breteler MM. Relation between smoking and risk of dementia and Alzheimer disease: the Rotterdam Study. *Neurology* 2007;69:998–1005.

104 Alonso A, Mosley THJ, Gottesman RF, *et al*. Risk of dementia hospitalisation associated with cardiovascular risk factors in midlife and older age: the Atherosclerosis Risk in Communities (ARIC) study. *Journal of Neurology, Neurosurgery, and Psychiatry* 2009;80:1194–201.

105 Rusanen M, Kivipelto M, Quesenberry CPJ, Zhou J, Whitmer RA. Heavy smoking in midlife and long-term risk of Alzheimer disease and vascular dementia. *Archives of Internal Medicine* 2011;171:333–9.

106 Rusanen M, Rovio S, Ngandu T, *et al*. Midlife smoking, apolipoprotein E and risk of dementia and Alzheimer's disease: a population-based cardiovascular risk factors, aging and dementia study. *Dementia and Geriatric Cognitive Disorders* 2010;30:277–84.

107 Cataldo JK, Prochaska JJ, Glantz SA. Cigarette smoking is a risk factor for Alzheimer's Disease: an analysis controlling for tobacco industry affiliation. *Journal of Alzheimer's Disease* 2010;19:465–80.

108 Iso H, Date C, Yamamoto A, *et al*. Perceived mental stress and mortality from cardiovascular disease among Japanese men and women: the Japan Collaborative Cohort

Study for Evaluation of Cancer Risk Sponsored by Monbusho (JACC Study). *Circulation* 2002;106:1229–36.

109 Carney CP, Woolson RF, Jones L, Noyes RJ, Doebbeling BN. Occurrence of cancer among people with mental health claims in an insured population. *Psychosomatic Medicine* 2004;66:735–43.

110 Albert CM, Chae CU, Rexrode KM, Manson JE, Kawachi I. Phobic anxiety and risk of coronary heart disease and sudden cardiac death among women. *Circulation* 2005;111:480–7.

111 Dalton SO, Mellemkjaer L, Thomassen L, Mortensen PB, Johansen C. Risk for cancer in a cohort of patients hospitalized for schizophrenia in Denmark, 1969–1993. *Schizophrenia Research* 2005;75:315–24.

112 Kroenke CH, Bennett GG, Fuchs C, *et al*. Depressive symptoms and prospective incidence of colorectal cancer in women. *American Journal of Epidemiology* 2005;162:839–48.

113 Hippisley-Cox J, Vinogradova Y, Coupland C, Parker C. Risk of malignancy in patients with schizophrenia or bipolar disorder: nested case-control study. *Archives of General Psychiatry* 2007;64:1368–76.

114 Goldacre MJ, Wotton CJ, Yeates D, Seagroatt V, Flint J. Cancer in people with depression or anxiety: record-linkage study. *Social Psychiatry and Psychiatric Epidemiology* 2007;42:683–9.

115 Mykletun A, Bjerkeset O, Dewey M, *et al*. Anxiety, depression, and cause-specific mortality: the HUNT study. *Psychosomatic Medicine* 2007;69:323–31.

116 Osborn DP, Levy G, Nazareth I, *et al*. Relative risk of cardiovascular and cancer mortality in people with severe mental illness from the United Kingdom's General Practice Research Database. *Archives of General Psychiatry* 2007;64:242–9.

117 Van der Kooy K, van Hout H, Marwijk H, *et al*. Depression and the risk for cardiovascular diseases: systematic review and meta analysis. *International Journal of Geriatric Psychiatry* 2007;22:613–26.

118 Catts VS, O'Toole BI, Frost AD. Cancer incidence in patients with schizophrenia and their first-degree relatives – a meta-analysis. *Acta Psychiatrica Scandinavica* 2008;117:323–36.

119 Nabi H, Hall M, Koskenvuo M, *et al*. Psychological and somatic symptoms of anxiety and risk of coronary heart disease: the health and social support prospective cohort study. *Biological Psychiatry* 2010;67:378–85.

120 Nabi H, Kivimäki M, Suominen S, *et al*. Does depression predict coronary heart disease and cerebrovascular disease equally well? The Health and Social Support Prospective Cohort Study. *International Journal of Epidemiology* 2010;39:1016–24.

121 Scherrer JF, Chrusciel T, Zeringue A, *et al*. Anxiety disorders increase risk for incident myocardial infarction in depressed and nondepressed Veterans Administration patients. *American Heart Journal* 2010;159:772–9.

122 Bresee LC, Majumdar SR, Patten SB, Johnson JA. Prevalence of cardiovascular risk factors and disease in people with schizophrenia: a population-based study. *Schizophrenia Research* 2010;117:75–82.

123 Melchior M, Ferrie JE, Alexanderson K, *et al*. Does sickness absence due to psychiatric disorder predict cause-specific mortality? A 16-year follow-up of the GAZEL occupational cohort study. *American Journal of Epidemiology* 2010;172:700–7.

124 Janszky I, Ahnve S, Lundberg I, Hemmingsson T. Early-onset depression, anxiety, and risk of subsequent coronary heart disease: 37-year follow-up of 49,321 young Swedish men. *Journal of the American College of Cardiology* 2010;56:31–7.

125 Ray WA, Meredith S, Thapa PB, *et al*. Antipsychotics and the risk of sudden cardiac death. *Archives of General Psychiatry* 2001;58:1161–7.

126 Penninx BW, Guralnik JM, Pahor M, *et al*. Chronically depressed mood and cancer risk in older persons. *Journal of the National Cancer Institute* 1998;90:1888–93.

5 Smoking cessation interventions for individuals with mental disorders

5.1 General considerations

Treatments for smokers typically comprise regular behavioural support combined with nicotine replacement therapy (NRT), or bupropion or varenicline pharmacotherapy. The effectiveness and cost-effectiveness of these interventions in the general population of smokers are well established and have been summarised in an extensive range of Cochrane systematic reviews[1–11] and guidance from the UK's National Institute for Health and Clinical Excellence (NICE).[12,13]

As discussed in earlier chapters, the occurrence of symptoms of mental disorders, especially anxiety and depression, is common in the UK, affecting almost one in four people at any time,[14] and smoking is particularly prevalent in this group. For various reasons, however, such as the common practice of excluding people with mental disorders from randomised trials of drug therapy[15] and the difficulty of recruiting and retaining people with severe mental illness (SMI) in clinical trials,[16] there is relatively little direct evidence on the effectiveness of smoking cessation interventions in people with mental disorders, eg a recent systematic review of smoking cessation in people with depression identified just 16 studies, only 3 of these recruiting smokers in whom depression was current.[17] As might be anticipated from the data on levels of dependence and perceived ability to quit smoking in Chapter 2, the efficacy of the cessation interventions in the studies included in the review was lower than in the general population of smokers, but the findings gave grounds to conclude that treatment strategies of proven effectiveness for the general population, particularly behavioural support and NRT, are also likely to be effective in people with common mental disorders.[17]

Addressing smoking in mental health settings, and particularly in secondary care, can pose major challenges, often exacerbated by a culture of acceptance of smoking. This historic culture is driven by various factors, including: the population norm of high smoking prevalence; assumptions that smoking constitutes a form of 'self-medication', the discontinuation of which would lead to exacerbation of symptoms of a mental disorder, or that people with mental disorders have little interest in stopping smoking or cannot successfully do so;

concerns that interventions effective in the general population are either not effective, or too difficult to use, or contraindicated in smokers with mental disorders; and use of tobacco as a means to build or control relationships between health professionals and patients.[18–23] These and other aspects of smoking cessation intervention in mental health secondary care settings will be addressed in detailed NICE guidance scheduled for publication later in 2013, but the management of smoking in the great majority of people with mental disorders, whose care is delivered outside the secondary care setting, remains an area of relative uncertainty.

However, the underlying mechanisms of addiction, and hence the principles of treating tobacco dependence, are common to all smokers and therefore provide a basis for treatment approaches that may simply need to be tailored to the special considerations for use in people with mental disorders. This chapter therefore addresses the application of smoking cessation and harm reduction interventions in people with mental disorders by drawing in particular on the available evidence for people with SMI provided by a recent (2010) systematic review of randomised controlled trials by Banham and Gilbody,[24] supplemented by reviews of treatment in schizophrenia by Tsoi *et al*[25,26] and other relevant studies published since 2010. The rationale adopted is that, in the absence of evidence to the contrary, smoking cessation interventions that are effective in the general population of smokers, and in people with SMI, are also likely to be so in those with the more common mental disorders. Examples of innovative approaches to improving service provision for people with mental disorders are also provided.

5.2 Cessation interventions for severe mental illness

Interventions evaluated in randomised controlled trials in people with SMI typically comprise specially designed individual or group behavioural programmes delivered in combination with pharmacotherapy, most commonly NRT and/or bupropion.[24] To date there has been little evidence published on the use of varenicline in this group.[27] Trials in SMI also tend not to involve long follow-up periods, so evidence for long-term efficacy is scarce. Evidence on cessation interventions in general, and specific considerations in SMI, are summarised in the following sections.

5.2.1 Behavioural support

In the general population, meta-analyses of trials comparing multi-session intensive behavioural support with brief advice have reported odds ratios (ORs) for cessation of 1.56 (95% confidence interval (CI) 1.32–1.84) for individual support, 2.04 (95% CI 1.60–2.60) for group support[5,6] and 1.64 (95% CI

1.41–1.92) for telephone support.[4] There is as yet insufficient information to determine which elements of behavioural support are effective, or whether one approach, such as motivational interviewing or cognitive–behavioural therapy, is more effective than another. However it appears that group support is generally more effective than one-to-one support, and that support should involve multiple sessions.[28]

In people with SMI, a study comparing a specialist quit smoking programme with standard smoking cessation group therapy, both delivered together with NRT,[29] found no difference in point prevalence abstinence at the primary trial endpoint of 3 months (relative risk (RR) of smoking = 1.01, 95% CI 0.45–2.28), although there was a non-significant reduction in smoking risk at the last time point of the study (8.5 months; RR = 0.61, 95% CI 0.14–2.67). Baker et al[30] compared the effectiveness of individual therapy (cognitive–behavioural therapy and motivational enhancement) plus NRT with usual care (booklets and access to primary care) without NRT among participants with SMI, predominantly schizophrenia. At 4 months (the trial endpoint), the intervention group were significantly more likely to abstain from smoking (RR = 2.74, 95% CI 1.10–6.81), although this effect was not sustained in later comparisons and the effect attributable to the behavioural intervention (as opposed to the NRT) is unclear. Thus, there is evidence that behavioural support delivered with NRT is effective in SMI, but no strong evidence that tailored behavioural interventions are more effective than standard group therapy.

5.2.2 Nicotine replacement therapy

A meta-analysis of more than 100 randomised controlled trials in general populations[9] has demonstrated that all forms of NRT (including transdermal patches, gum, inhalator, nasal spray, lozenges and others) are similarly effective in aiding long-term cessation (overall OR 1.77, 95% CI 1.66–1.88), and that combinations of slower (transdermal patches) and faster-acting NRT formulations (oral or nasal delivery products) are more effective than either formulation alone.

Use of NRT in people with SMI has not been subject to large-scale clinical trials, although there are no grounds to suspect that NRT is likely to be ineffective in this population. However, smokers with SMI tend to smoke more cigarettes,[31,32] and to smoke each cigarette more intensely and hence extract more nicotine from each cigarette,[33] so the severity of nicotine withdrawal symptoms is likely to be particularly intense in this group. As in the general population of more dependent smokers, it is therefore probably especially important to use combination NRT,[9] supplementing a transdermal patch with a faster-acting product (of which the nasal spray may be particularly effective[34]), in people with SMI. It is also probably important to continue NRT for longer than the typically recommended 8–12 weeks, and indeed to consider long-term nicotine substitution as a harm reduction strategy for people who experience difficulty with nicotine withdrawal (see section 5.3)

5.2.3 Bupropion

In general population studies, bupropion is similarly effective to single-formulation NRT for smoking cessation, with a pooled RR relative to placebo of 1.69 (95% CI 1.53–1.85).[2] For people with SMI, in three trials comparing bupropion with placebo, delivered with group therapy,[35–37] meta-analysis confirmed strong and significant superiority of treatment with bupropion at trial endpoints (RR = 4.18, 95% CI 1.30–13.42).[24] Effectiveness was also demonstrated in two trials comparing a bupropion/NRT combination with NRT only, delivered together with group therapy,[38,39] with an RR for cessation of 2.34 (95% CI 1.12–4.91).[24] A Cochrane review of bupropion effectiveness in people with schizophrenia,[25] involving seven trials, estimated a pooled RR of cessation of 2.78 (95% CI 1.02–7.58), with no reported serious adverse events.[26]

The primary adverse effect of bupropion is an increased risk of seizures, so bupropion should be used with particular caution together with other medications used in SMI, including tricyclic antidepressants and some antipsychotic agents, which also lower the seizure threshold. Bupropion is contraindicated in bipolar affective disorder because it is an antidepressant and hence theoretically poses a risk of precipitating mania. Other cautions on bupropion use are summarised in section 5.2.5.

5.2.4 Varenicline

The nicotine receptor partial agonist varenicline is probably the most effective cessation pharmacotherapy in the general population of smokers (summary OR for 12-month continuous abstinence for varenicline relative to placebo = 3.22, 95% CI 2.43–4.27).[1] It is more effective in cessation trials than bupropion (OR for varenicline vs bupropion = 1.66, 95% CI 1.28–2.16).[1] To date, however, evidence on the effectiveness of varenicline in people with mental disorders is particularly limited, in large part because of early concerns that varenicline may lead to the exacerbation of symptoms, especially depression, and induce thoughts of self-harm and suicide. Although a large UK primary care epidemiological study in the general population of smokers has reported that these serious adverse events are generally rare in people who use medication to quit smoking, and are not statistically significantly more common with varenicline, modest increases in risk of adverse events, which may be particularly relevant to those with mental disorders, could not be ruled out.[40]

In people with SMI, a recent randomised trial conducted in the USA,[41] and a review of case and pilot studies on the efficacy and tolerability of varenicline in smokers with schizophrenia, indicate that varenicline is effective but recommend careful supervision and monitoring for exacerbation of psychiatric symptoms.[27] In terms of effectiveness this evidence is promising: the 12-week, randomised, double-blind, multicenter US trial, in which 84 patients received varenicline and 43 placebo, found abstinence rates of 19% versus 4.7% at 12 weeks, and 11.9% versus 2.3% at 24 weeks.[41] Other available evidence, although limited, provides further support: a 12-week, open-label, smoking cessation trial of varenicline combined with weekly group cognitive–behavioural therapy in 112 stable outpatients with schizophrenia[42] found 2-week and 4-week continuous abstinence rates of 47.3% and of 34% respectively, and significant reductions in smoking (measured by exhaled carbon monoxide) in those who did not succeed in quitting. A pilot study in eight outpatients with schizophrenia or schizoaffective disorder,[43] randomised to varenicline (1 mg twice a day) or placebo for 12 weeks delivered together with individual behavioural support, found that three of four participants treated with varenicline achieved continuous abstinence (weeks 8–12, verified with expired CO), compared with no participant in the placebo group. Smith *et al*,[44] in a study of 14 smokers with schizophrenia, found that treatment with varenicline led to some cognitive improvement, as well as to smoking reduction and reduced CO expired and cotinine levels.

In a multicentre randomised trial of varenicline in over 500 smokers with major depression, reported at the time of writing only in a press statement, 4-week continuous abstinence rates at 3 months were 35.9% in those receiving varenicline, compared with 15.6% of participants receiving placebo, and 20.3% and 10.4% respectively at 1 year.[45] The study is reported to have found no difference in adverse events between treatment groups, although detailed comparisons are not provided.[45] Further randomised trials and surveillance data on use of varenicline in people with mental disorders are urgently required, but the available evidence suggests that, with careful supervision and monitoring, varenicline is likely to be safe and effective in this group.

5.2.5 Cautions on use of bupropion and varenicline

In view of concerns over the occurrence of depression, suicidal thoughts, suicide attempts and completed suicides in patients taking varenicline, and updates from the Medicines and Healthcare products Regulatory Agency[46] and the US Food and Drug Administration (FDA),[47] current guidance from The Royal College of General Practitioners (RCGP) and The Royal College of Psychiatrists[31] in the UK recommends that both varenicline and bupropion be used under close, coordinated supervision by health professionals, especially in the first 2–3 weeks of therapy, that family members and caregivers be alerted to the potential for adverse effects, and that varenicline or bupropion be discontinued immediately in the event of any cause for concern.

5.3 Cutting down on smoking, and other harm reduction strategies

Promoting smoking reduction as an option for those who do not wish to attempt abrupt cessation has been controversial due to concerns that cutting down may provide false reassurance of reduced hazard, and perpetuate smoking by postponing a definitive quit attempt. For various reasons, including heavier smoking of the reduced number of cigarettes (compensation) and the exposure–response relationships between smoking and disease, the health benefits accrued from cutting down are likely to be disproportionately low in relation to reductions in the number of cigarettes smoked. A recent systematic review concluded that a substantial reduction in smoking seems to have a modest health benefit, although the long-term effects of smoking reduction are uncertain.[48]

However, smoking reduction does yield substantial benefits in the general population by increasing the likelihood of a definitive quit attempt in the future.[49,50] Encouraging smokers to use NRT to cut down on smoking without a commitment to quit doubles the likelihood of a successful quit attempt.[51] Harm reduction strategies,[52] by which people who are otherwise unlikely or unwilling to quit are encouraged to substitute smoked tobacco with alternative sources of nicotine for long-term use, therefore offer substantial potential to prevent harm from smoking by both directly reducing the amount of smoke inhaled and making complete cessation more likely. This approach, which in addition to NRT embraces the potential of substitution using alternative nicotine devices such as electronic cigarettes, is endorsed in draft guidance from NICE[53] due for final publication in May 2013. Given the high levels of dependence on smoking and low perceived likelihood of quitting outlined in Chapter 2, harm reduction has evident major potential as a means to promote smoking cessation, and support smoke-free policies, in mental health settings. This potential is to date highly under-researched, and evidence on the effectiveness of harm reduction in SMI is currently limited, however, to analyses of secondary outcomes in a heterogeneous range of cessation studies[35–38,54,55] summarised in the following sections.

5.3.1 Behavioural interventions

A study of a specialist smoking programme for SMI comprising 3 weeks of motivational enhancement therapy and 7 weeks of psychoeducation, social skills and relapse prevention training, compared with standard group therapy to achieve reductions in the numbers of cigarettes smoked, reported no difference in change in mean exhaled CO relative to baseline over 3 months.[29] This suggests that any reduction in cigarette consumption (which was not reported in the study) had been counterbalanced by compensatory smoking. Cigarette consumption was reduced, however, in a study of eight sessions of motivational interviewing and cognitive–behavioural therapy, which increased the likelihood of a 50% reduction in consumption by a ratio of 2.62 (95% CI 1.76–3.93) at 4 months and 1.75 (95% CI 1.15–2.66) at 13 months.[30]

5.3.2 Nicotine replacement therapy

In a study of 10 participants with schizophrenia, Dalack and Meador-Woodruff[54] reported modest but non-significant reductions in mean expired CO after short-term use of NRT.

5.3.3 Bupropion

Two studies have reported significant reductions in mean CO levels and numbers of cigarettes smoked at up to 3 months after receiving group therapy plus bupropion, relative to group therapy alone.[36,37] Another reported significant reductions in mean serum cotinine levels during, but not after, treatment.[35] A study using bupropion with NRT reported a significant increase in the likelihood of achieving self-reported 7-day smoking reduction of 50% or more, and CO reduction of 40% or more after 3 months (RR 1.95; 95% CI 1.01–3.77), although not at earlier endpoints.[38]

5.3.4 Varenicline

Evidence on the effectiveness of varenicline for smoking reduction is scarce, and to our knowledge is limited to an uncontrolled before and after study in 14 men with schizophrenia or schizoaffective disorder, most of whom did not express strong motivation to stop smoking. This study reported a non-significant reduction in the average number of cigarettes smoked per day, from 36.5 to 12.5, when treated with varenicline (mean, $p = 0.12$).[44] Significant reductions were also observed in expired CO (from a mean of 9 ppm (parts per million) before to 5 ppm after) and plasma cotinine levels (from 239 ng/mL before to 130 ng/mL after).

5.4 Is it safe for people with SMI to give up smoking?

Many mental health professionals are concerned that smoking cessation may impact adversely on mental health, and this perception can pose a barrier to the implementation of smoking cessation interventions in mental health settings.[18,20,22,56] This is a serious concern which, if grounded in fact, might add some legitimacy to continued use of tobacco in this population. We summarise the evidence on adverse events, psychological wellbeing and other consequences of smoking cessation in people with SMI in the following sections.

5.4.1 Adverse events relating to smoking cessation interventions

Evidence on adverse events occurring in the context of stopping smoking aided by different pharmacological regimens suggests that, overall, smoking cessation interventions in people with mental disorders are well tolerated and safe. Of four studies in people with schizophrenia exploring adverse events with bupropion alone or in combination with NRT in people with schizophrenia, two used the Systematic Assessment For Treatment Emergent Effects (SAFTEE),[35,36] and two recorded events descriptively.[38,39] In placebo-controlled studies of bupropion, no adverse events were reported in the smallest, involving 18 participants,[35] whereas a study involving 53 participants reported three adverse events requiring trial withdrawal: one a probable medication allergy, and two cases of suicidal ideation (trial group not clear).[36] A study of 51 patients with schizophrenia using bupropion or placebo in addition to NRT[38] reported four trial withdrawals due to medication side effects, two in the intervention group, whereas a similar study by George *et al*[39] reported three serious adverse events described as psychotic decompensation, two of which occurred in the placebo group.

Adverse events relating to the concurrent use of NRT while smoking were assessed in a study of smoking reduction;[54] none were reported. For varenicline, the available evidence[27,41,45] suggests that the medication is well tolerated in participants with schizophrenia, schizoaffective disorders and major depression, with no differences in the occurrence of adverse events detected between the respective intervention and placebo groups; however, side effects in the form of nausea and insomnia are common, as is the case with this drug in the general population. A study conducted in the military health service in the USA showed that there does not appear to be an increase in neuropsychiatric hospitalisations with varenicline compared with NRT patch over 30 or 60 days after drug initiation.[57]

5.4.2 Effects of smoking cessation on mental health symptoms

Studies using validated symptom scales to ascertain whether psychiatric symptoms change during cessation interventions generally suggest that smoking cessation has no negative impact on psychiatric symptoms in people with schizophrenia, and that there may in fact be benefits in relation to depression and anxiety, eg in patients with schizophrenia receiving cessation interventions significantly lower scores have been reported on the Beck Depression Index II (BDI-II), Short Form 12 (SF-12) and State Trait Anxiety Inventory (STAI),[30] reduced Brief Psychiatric Rating Scale (BPRS) general score,[35] improved Positive and Negative Symptoms Scale (PANSS) scores,[36] and lower Barnes Akathisia Scale and Simpson Angus Scale (SAS) scores for extrapyramidal side effects,[38] and a greater decrease in PANSS score (negative symptoms).[39] A recent study of

491 NHS stop smoking service (NHS SSS) users also showed that those succeeding at a quit attempt experienced a marked reduction in anxiety symptoms compared with baseline, thus contradicting the common assumption that smoking is a stress reliever.[58]

5.4.3 Weight gain

Weight gain can be a significant problem among people with SMI, and reflects prevalent dietary patterns, low exercise levels and side effects of some medications. Concerns about additional weight gain resulting from quitting smoking are relevant in the general population[59] and especially so among smokers with SMI.[60] In the general population, smoking cessation is typically associated with a gain in weight of 5 kg or more relative to those who continue to smoke, and more in those who are already overweight. Similar outcomes might be expected in people with SMI, although the randomised trial literature on effects in SMI is not especially informative on this outcome; we are aware of only one study that has reported change in weight in participants with SMI, which reported no increase.[35]

5.4.4 Interactions with treatment for mental disorders

Metabolism of several psychotropic drugs is increased in cigarette smokers. This effect is not due to nicotine, but to inhaled polycyclic aromatic hydrocarbons in smoke, which induce cytochrome P450 (CYP) CYP1A2 isoenzymes[61] to metabolise many commonly used antipsychotics and antidepressants more quickly. Patients who smoke are therefore likely to need higher doses of these drugs to achieve similar blood levels to non-smokers, and in the event of stopping smoking need to reduce the doses used to compensate for this effect. This applies in particular to clozapine and olanzapine, two commonly used antipsychotic medications metabolised primarily by CYP1A2,[62] and pharmacokinetic studies have demonstrated more rapid clearance of olanzapine and lower clozapine concentrations in participants who smoke compared with those who don't.[63,64] Adverse clinical outcomes arising from rapid increases in blood levels of these drugs after stopping smoking have been reported,[65,66] with symptoms including somnolence, hypersalivation, fatigue, extrapyramidal effects, delirium and seizures.[65,67] Clinical guidelines recommend reducing doses of these drugs by around 25% during the first week after stopping smoking, and monitoring blood levels before and at weekly intervals after stopping smoking until levels have stabilised.[68] Similar considerations apply to a range of other psychotropic drugs, for which recommendations are given in Table 5.1.

Nicotine is metabolised predominantly by a different CYP enzyme, CYP2A6, which is induced by oral contraceptive medications and carbamazepine.[61,69]

Table 5.1 Prescribing guidelines for psychotropic drugs in smoking cessation[68]

Drug	Effect of smoking	Action to be taken on stopping smoking	Action to be taken on smoking relapse
Benzodiazepines	Plasma levels reduced by 0–50% (depends on drug and smoking status)	Monitor closely. Consider reducing dose by up to 25% over one week	Monitor closely. Consider restarting 'normal' smoking dose
Carbamazepine	Unclear, but smoking may reduce carbamazepine plasma levels to a small extent	Monitor for changes in severity of adverse effects	Monitor plasma levels
Chlorpromazine	Plasma levels reduced. Varied estimates of exact effect	Monitor closely, consider dose reduction	Monitor closely, consider restarting previous smoking dose
Clozapine	Reduces plasma levels by up to 50%. Plasma level reduction may be greater in those receiving valporate	Take plasma level before stopping. On stopping, reduce dose gradually (over a week) until around 75% of original dose reached (ie reduce by 25%). Repeat plasma level one week after stopping. Consider further dose reductions	Take plasma level before restarting. Increase dose to previous smoking dose over one week. Repeat plasma level
Duloxetine	Plasma levels may be reduced by up to 50%	Monitor closely. Dose may need to be reduced	Consider re-introducing previous smoking dose

continued

Table 5.1 continued

Drug	Effect of smoking	Action to be taken on stopping smoking	Action to be taken on smoking relapse
Fluphenazine	Reduces plasma levels by up to 50%	On stopping, reduce dose by 25%. Monitor carefully over following 4–8 weeks. Consider further dose reductions.	On restarting, increase dose to previous dose
Fluvoxamine	Plasma levels decreased by around a third	Monitor closely. Dose may need to be reduced	Dose may need to be increased to previous level
Haloperidol	Reduces plasma levels by around 20%	Reduce dose by around 10%. Monitor carefully. Consider further dose reductions	On restarting, increase dose to previous dose
Mirtzapine	Unclear, but effect probably minimal	Monitor	Monitor
Olanzapine	Reduces plasma levels by up to 50%	Take plasma level before stopping. On stopping, reduce dose by 25%. After one week, repeat plasma level. Consider further dose reductions	Take plasma level before restarting. Increase dose to previous smoking dose over one week. Repeat plasma level
Tricyclic antidepressants	Plasma levels reduced by 25–50%	Monitor closely. Consider reducing the dose by 10–25% over one week. Consider further dose reductions	Monitor closely. Consider restarting previous smoking dose
Zuclopentixol	Unclear, but effect probably minimal	Monitor	Monitor

Smokers using these drugs would be expected to compensate their intake of nicotine from cigarettes to maintain blood levels, but starting these drugs in smokers using NRT for smoking cessation or abstinence is likely to reduce the efficacy of the NRT. Nicotine is not known to have any clinically significant interactions with other medications.

5.4.5 Interactions with caffeine

Caffeine is also metabolised by CYP1A2, up to 60–70% faster in smokers than non-smokers,[61] and is one probable reason why cigarette smokers tend to drink more coffee than non-smokers.[69] Caffeine metabolism decreases within 3 or 4 days of stopping smoking and, if coffee consumption continues unchanged, can lead to symptoms including agitation, irritability or poor concentration which can be confused with or exacerbate symptoms of both nicotine withdrawal and mental disorders. High caffeine levels persist weeks or months after quitting smoking.[70] People who smoke, particularly those with high caffeine intakes, should therefore be advised to reduce caffeine when they quit smoking; this may be particularly important for smokers with schizophrenia, among whom very high serum caffeine levels have been reported.[71]

5.4.6 Nicotine withdrawal symptoms

Abrupt cessation or reduction in nicotine use in people who smoke regularly results in symptoms of nicotine withdrawal, which can include dysphoric or depressed mood, insomnia, irritability, frustration, anger, anxiety, difficulty concentrating and restlessness.[72] These symptoms tend to be more severe in smokers with SMI,[73–76] and their non-specificity can result in misattribution to mental disorders and inappropriate treatment responses. A study of smokers with schizophrenia admitted to a smoke-free hospital found higher levels of agitation in those with greater nicotine dependence, and a significant reduction in agitation in those who received a 21 mg nicotine patch relative to a placebo.[77] It is therefore particularly important to ensure that adequate doses of NRT are provided to people with mental disorders who smoke during quit attempts or other abstention from smoking.

5.4.7 Effects of antipsychotic medication on smoking cessation

Antipsychotic medication can also influence smoking behaviour. Smokers using 'atypical' antipsychotics such as clozapine, as opposed to first-generation ('typical') treatments such as haloperidol, are more likely to quit smoking.[29] Clozapine treatment is also associated with reduced smoking, particularly in heavy smokers and in those showing a therapeutic response to clozapine.[78–80] Clozapine is the only atypical antipsychotic that consistently improves P50 auditory gating, probably through serotonin ($5HT_3$) receptor antagonism, which increases acetylcholine release,[81] and hence activates nicotinic receptors which reduce the desire to smoke. Conversely, treatment with the older typical antipsychotics, such as haloperidol, has been associated with increased smoking.[79]

5.5 Provision of smoking cessation and tobacco dependence treatment for smokers with mental disorders in the UK

The UK government's mental health strategy *(No health without mental health)* has recently highlighted the need to adress the current higher mortality, lower levels of general health, and lower uptake of mainstream screening and public health programmes by people with mental disorders.[82] The identification of smokers with mental disorders, and provision of support to stop smoking through improved access to appropriate smoking cessation programmes, are described as critical objectives.[82] Smokers with mental disorders can access smoking cessation treatment services through a variety of avenues including their general (primary care) practitioner (GP), services provided by mental health trusts and by self-enrolment with a local NHS SSS. These services, and the challenges that they present, are outlined below.

5.5.1 Primary care

As most people with mental disorders are managed in primary care, the role of the GP in providing smoking cessation and harm reduction treatment is crucial. This has recently been acknowledged in the integration of mental health-specific smoking-related outcomes into the Quality of Outcomes Framework (QOF),[83] which is used to measure and incentivise GPs' performance in the UK. The new indicators reward GPs for documenting smoking status regularly in patients with schizophrenia, bipolar disorder and other psychoses, and for providing smoking cessation advice or referral to an NHS SSS.[83] For the general population, brief advice by a practitioner, defined as the provision of 'verbal instructions to stop smoking with or without added information about the harmful effects of smoking', and requiring only 1 or 2 minutes of consultation time, achieves modest effects but is highly cost-effective.[84] Success can be increased by around 40% if more intensive advice is given with reinforcement by CO reading.[84] Although research into the effectiveness of brief and intensive advice for populations with mental disorders alone is lacking, there is no reason to believe that it would not achieve modest success in people with mental disorders, particularly if supported by appropriate prescribing of cessation pharmacotherapy.

Although data from the USA suggest that, in the past, primary care physicians (and indeed many other health professionals) have failed to address[85] or even tacitly encourage smoking, for reasons related to common beliefs and perceptions in terms of its therapeutic value and the risks of cessation for patients' mental health ('first things first'; see also sections 5.1 and 6.3), the data in Chapter 2 suggest that, in the UK at least, practice is changing. The revised QOF is likely to have contributed substantially to this, at least in the patient groups specified in the QOF (schizophrenia, bipolar disorder or other psychoses). It is important, however, to ensure that this intervention is delivered to maximum effect and that all smokers, irrespective of co-morbidity, are offered and delivered the maximum level of intervention that they are willing to accept. In line with new NICE guidance,[53] it is also important that smokers who decline help to quit smoking are encouraged to adopt harm reduction strategies.

5.5.2 Specialist mental health settings (secondary care)

Specialist inpatient and community mental health services, provided by NHS mental health trusts, should be able to play major roles in addressing smoking, at several levels.

First, people with severe mental disorders, many of whom do not access mainstream services (including primary care) regularly, will be in regular contact with these services in the context of the care programme approach, which stipulates the development of a care plan, the identification of a 'care coordinator' and an annual review by a consultant psychiatrist.[86] Smoking cessation should be a prominent part of this wider care delivery, in accordance with mental health strategy objectives.[82]

Second, there is now clear evidence that patients admitted to inpatient wards tend to change their smoking behaviour by decreasing, increasing or even starting to smoke,[87,88] possibly as a consequence of adapting to inpatient routines and smoking breaks (see Chapter 6, section 6.2). Admission is, however, an opportunity to intervene to reduce smoking,[89] particularly in the context of strong smoke-free policies in British settings. Motivation to stop smoking is similarly high in hospitalised patients with and without a mental disorder,[90] and a Cochrane review of smoking cessation interventions for hospitalised patients found that intensive counselling interventions started during admission and continued for at least 1 month after discharge increased cessation rates (OR = 1.65, 95% CI 1.44–1.90; 17 trials) regardless of admission diagnosis.[15]

Third, specialist mental health services are particularly suitable settings in which to provide tailored support through experienced mental health staff, in environments and contexts familiar to service users and with appropriate attention to treatment interactions, and with recognition and appropriate attribution of withdrawal symptoms.

Fourth, active promotion of a smoke-free lifestyle should also be an integral part of any health service, including those for mental disorders.

Finally, nicotine substitution as a harm reduction strategy and/or to enable compliance with smoke-free environments in secondary care settings should be a default support for smokers unwilling or otherwise unable to engage in cessation activities but obliged by admission to a smoke-free setting to abstain from smoking.

However, there is little available information on the extent to which stop smoking support is (or is not) delivered within specialist mental health settings in England. Although all NHS mental health trusts in England have now implemented smoke-free policies, most of which are likely to include a statement on the importance of addressing smoking and providing appropriate support or referrals to NHS SSS, in the absence of minimum standards, reporting requirements or monitoring in this area makes it difficult to evaluate the effectiveness of these policies. Overall, there is evidence that resources allocated to enforcing smoke-free policies, including those that would ensure the provision of adequate behavioural and pharmacological support (such as staff training and provision of NRT), are often lacking and that complex barriers to the implementation of effective tobacco dependence treatment in mental healthcare settings exist.[21,22,91] Perhaps most fundamentally, studies have highlighted how the 'culture' within mental healthcare settings tends to facilitate smoking[19] (see Chapter 6, section 6.2 for details).

A possible vehicle for implementation of more systematic delivery of stop smoking support in mental health settings is the Commissioning for Quality and Innovation (CQUIN) payment framework,[83] which was introduced in 2009 as a national framework for locally agreed priorities; it was intended for use by commissioners to reward excellence by linking a proportion of providers' income to the achievement of local quality improvement goals. The focus of the framework on innovation and directly measurable indicators that are aligned with national priorities would seem to suggest stop smoking support programmes within mental health settings as an ideal application for CQUIN schemes. However, as the schemes are negotiated locally, there is no currently agreed standard for this.

5.5.3 Child and adolescent mental health services

As most smoking starts before adulthood, prevention of uptake among adolescent non-smokers and intervention to promote cessation in young people who smoke are especially important. A recent meta-analysis has demonstrated that smoking prevalence among young people at the time of presentation for treatment of first-episode psychosis is around 60%, and six times higher than in age- and gender-matched controls,[92] demonstrating that more attention needs to be paid to the reasons for starting tobacco use before diagnosis, as well as exploring better ways to help smokers quit. However, there is no evidence available on provision and/or effect of tobacco dependence treatment in child and adolescent mental health service (CAMHS) settings in the UK. The lack of research in this area is counterintuitive to its obvious importance and clearly highlights the need for future initiatives.

5.5.4 NHS stop smoking services

In 1998 in the UK, the White Paper *Smoking Kills* announced new government funding to set up what have become known as NHS SSS.[93] Originally focused in areas of socioeconomic deprivation, the aim was to apply cessation services as a mechanism to reduce health inequality. Within a few years, however, almost every primary care trust area had established a dedicated NHS SSS, and in 2009–10 the services helped over three-quarters of a million smokers to make a quit attempt.[94] NHS SSS treatment usually comprises several weekly behavioural support sessions supplemented by NRT, or varenicline or bupropion pharmacotherapy (see section 5.1). The behavioural support is led by a trained stop smoking practitioner and delivered either individually or in a group-based format. Increasingly, a range of health professionals collaborates with the specialist SSS in the delivery of support (including those in both primary and secondary care).[94]

As outlined in section 5.1, there is no reason why the treatment programmes delivered by NHS SSS should not be appropriate for most people living with a mental disorder, particularly if adapted to meet the special demands and high levels of dependence prevalent in this group. However, a recent survey suggests that only a minority of NHS SSS routinely assess the mental health status or mental health service use of their clients, and that most services do not routinely implement special checks or actions even if mental health problems are revealed.[95] As SSS audit work has shown that at least one in nine clients of NHS SSS has a current and diagnosed mental health condition,[96] the need for widespread adoption of appropriate protocols within these services is evident. Towards this aim, the most recent national guidance aimed at NHS SSS[97] includes full guidance on treating people with mental disorders. Furthermore, the National Centre for Smoking Cessation and Treatment has recently developed a specialist module to train smoking cessation advisers on the specific links between smoking and mental illness.

NHS SSS have been shown to be highly cost-effective, the average cost per life gained being as low as £684.[98] However, it has been argued that the system within which such services operate may prevent them from fulfilling their full potential to reduce health inequalities,[99] in particular because services have traditionally been driven by large quantitative '4-week' quit targets. The demands of these targets have to date tended to inhibit provision of services for people, including those with mental health problems, who are disadvantaged and may require more resource-intensive support.[99] SSS also need to be equally available to patients in secondary care or other health settings in which access to community-based services is limited or impractical.

5.5.5 Enhancing service provision for smokers with mental disorders

It is evident that much could be done to improve smoking cessation service provision for people with mental disorders in the future. Recent government strategies and service guidance reflect this; the mental health strategy highlights that closer working between primary and mental health secondary care staff would facilitate integration of tobacco dependence support across treatment settings, and help support the confidence of mental health staff to identify and intervene in smoking and other adverse health behaviours. Revised service and monitoring guidance for NHS SSS also emphasises the importance of targeting and supporting people with mental disorders, and recommends improved coordination between NHS SSS and primary care, community and acute mental health services. It specifically states that health inequalities experienced by people with mental disorders will widen if investment in smoking cessation for this group is not greater than for the general population.

Thus, the development of suitable incentives for service providers (such as smoking-related QOF outcomes for GPs and potentially CQUIN targets for mental health trusts) and the development of guidance for the delivery of adequately tailored treatment for certain groups of people with mental disorders (notably those with severe and enduring illness) are likely to support the enhancement of service provision in the future.

5.6 Experience of attempts to introduce comprehensive smoking cessation support in mental health settings: UK case studies

5.6.1 London, UK

A 3-year project (2008–11), funded jointly by Merton Borough Local Authority and South-West London and St George's Mental Health Trust, aimed to develop a defined pathway of smoking treatment for mental health service users by training all frontline staff to identify all smokers and deliver brief advice to quit, and to refer smokers to a specialist adviser based in inpatient or community clinics and employed to deliver stop smoking support[100] (Fig 5.1). The adviser provided a structured behavioural support programme and combination NRT in accordance with NICE guidance.[12] Face-to-face behavioural support was provided for at least 12 weeks, whereas smokers were encouraged to cut down their smoking in advance of a chosen quit date, and received continued support

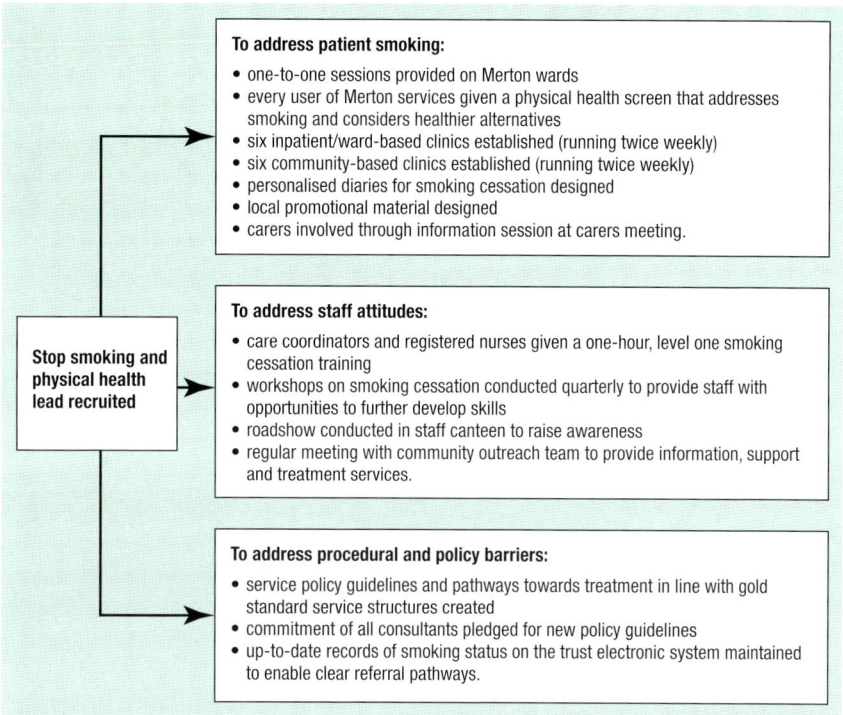

Fig 5.1 Steps along the smoking treatment pathway.

for up to 4 weeks thereafter. Over 400 healthcare professionals (95% of frontline staff) were trained to deliver interventions, and 180 patients accessed the service, most of whom achieved assisted reduction. The number of patients successfully quitting per quarter totalled 38 after 18 months of the specialist adviser being in post. The greatest challenges were perceived to be related to staff attitudes reflecting reluctant engagement with smoking cessation interventions for patients with SMI, and to the development of adequate pathways including prescriptions and management of pharmacotherapy.

5.6.2 Nottingham, UK

This project, part of a series of pilot projects funded by the Department of Health to address tobacco-related inequalities, aimed to develop, implement and appraise a tailored tobacco dependence service in mental health settings[101] (Fig 5.2). It also aimed to address barriers to sustainable implementation by addressing knowledge gaps, common misconceptions and more complex systemic issues relating to the 'smoking culture' in mental health settings, to develop instruments and materials suitable to be integrated in care pathways, and to improve collaboration with the local NHS SSS in the context of an integrative service model. The project was

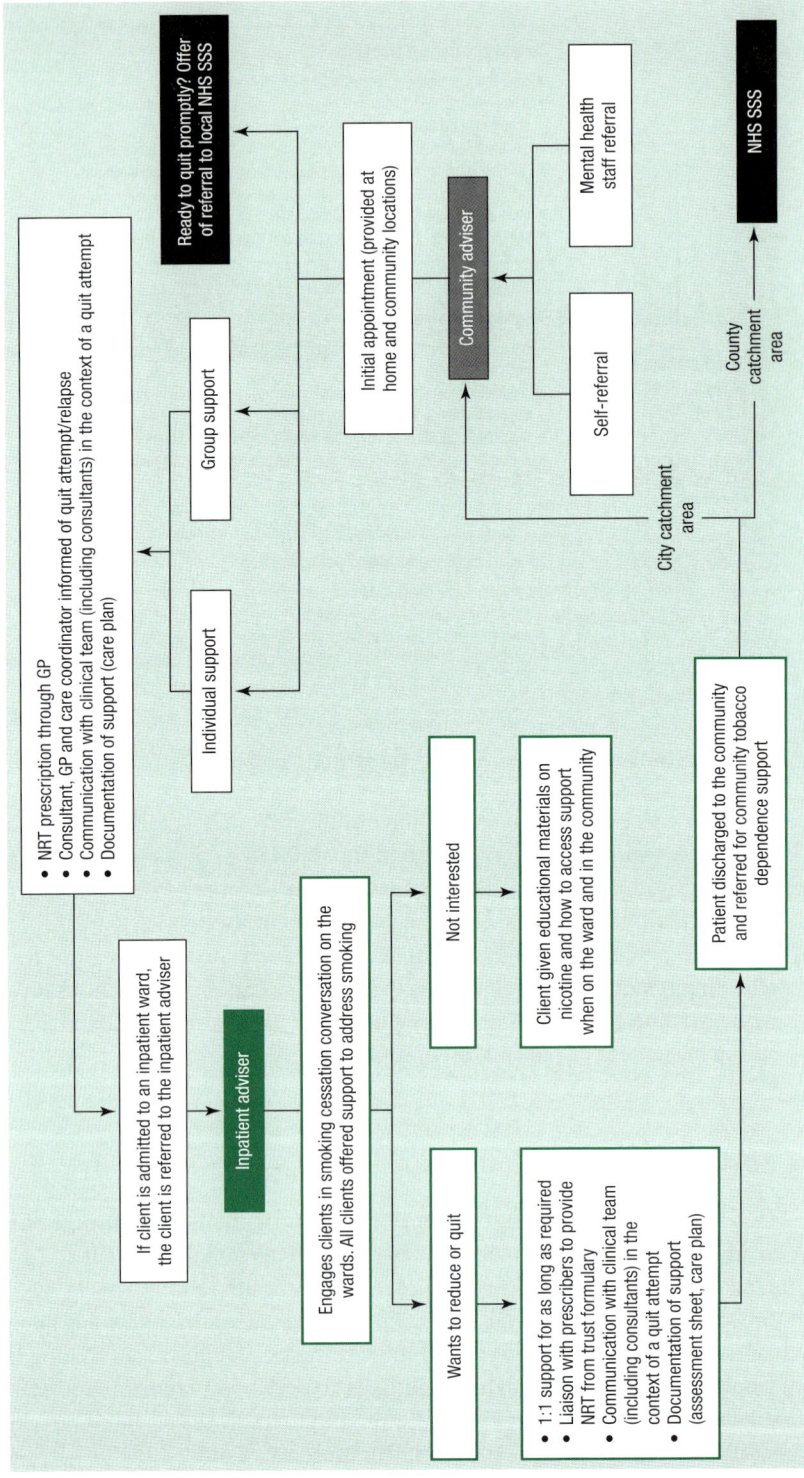

Fig 5.2 Structure of Nottingham tobacco dependence support service. NRT, nicotine replacement therapy; SSS, stop smoking services.

carried out on two acute adult mental health wards and two rehabilitation wards (129 beds), and in a community recovery team caring for over 2000 patients, between October 2010 and June 2011. Two mental health professionals were trained in tobacco dependence and employed full time to support patient and staff smokers in the project settings, to deliver staff training and involve staff in service provision, and to develop instruments and materials central to the provision of comprehensive support in collaboration with the project team. Instruments for the integration of smoking treatment into care pathways, such as assessment sheets, tobacco dependence treatment plans and guidance related to potentially necessary adjustment of antipsychotic dosage, as well as comprehensive communication structures between all treatment providers (including GPs), were developed. A referral system to the local NHS SSS was also created.

By the end of this project, 110 patients, comprising 53 inpatients (23% of all inpatient smokers) and 57 community patients (of an unknown number of community smokers, because recording of smoking status was not mandatory in this setting), had attended at least one support session with a specialist adviser. Of those, 34 (31%) had made a quit attempt and 17 (50% of those trying) had successfully quit by the final contact. A further 29 patients (26%) reduced cigarette consumption by up to 50% at the final contact. Barriers to service implementation were complex and mainly related to the following themes: (1) trust policy, systems and procedures, (2) staff knowledge and attitudes, and (3) illness-related factors.

5.6.3 Implications for practice

These case studies indicate at best modest success of tailored tobacco dependence support services in terms of absolute numbers of successful quit attempts, but reflect a general interest in and demand for support. They also suggest the existence of a discrepancy between outcomes of efficacy studies conducted in controlled study settings (see section 5.1), and those following the translation of the evidence base into practice. To develop and deliver tailored, 'workable' support models in mental health settings successfully, complex systemic barriers remain to be addressed, even in a country with a strong anti-smoking climate such as the UK. These include addressing staff knowledge, attitudes and behaviour related to smoking (including staff smoking) and the development-related information, and providing appropriate support.

5.7 Summary

> - Smoking cessation interventions that combine behavioural support with cessation pharmacotherapy, and are effective in the general population, are also likely to be effective in people with mental disorders.

- NRT is effective in people with mental disorders, but is likely to be required in high doses, for longer durations and with more intensive behavioural support than in the general population of smokers.
- Bupropion and varenicline are both effective in people with mental disorders, but should be used with appropriate supervision and monitoring; further research on their use in this population is an urgent priority.
- Smoking cessation does not exacerbate symptoms of mental disorders, and improves symptoms in the longer term.
- However, symptoms of nicotine withdrawal are easily confused with those of underlying mental disorder, and should be treated with NRT or other cessation therapy.
- Smoking cessation reduces the metabolism of some drugs, such as clozapine, used to treat mental disorder, necessitating prompt reduction in doses of affected drugs at the time of quitting, and increases in the event of relapse.
- Smokers who do not want to quit smoking, or else feel unable to make a quit attempt, should be encouraged to cut down on smoking, and to use NRT or other nicotine-containing devices (in line with NICE tobacco harm reduction guidance) to support smoking abstinence in secondary care or other smoke-free settings, and promote the likelihood of future quit attempts.
- All primary and secondary care services should record smoking status and provide effective cessation or harm reduction interventions as a central, systematic component of care delivery. Where access to community-based services is limited, as, for example, in secondary care settings, services should be provided in-house.
- As many people with mental disorders are managed by both primary and secondary care, provision of smoking cessation support in primary and secondary care settings requires coordination to ensure consistency.
- Further research is urgently required to improve the design and content of cessation and harm reduction interventions in mental health settings, and to maximise access to and delivery of evidence-based support.

References

1 Cahill K, Stead LF, Lancaster T. Nicotine receptor partial agonists for smoking cessation. *Cochrane Database of Systematic Reviews* 2007;(4):CD006103.

2 Hughes JR, Stead LF, Lancaster T. Antidepressants for smoking cessation. *Cochrane Database of Systematic Reviews* 2007;(1):CD000031.

3 Lancaster T, Stead LF. Physician advice for smoking cessation. *Cochrane Database of Systematic Reviews* 2004;(4):CD000165.

4 Lancaster T, Perera R, Stead LF. Telephone counselling for smoking cessation. *Cochrane Database of Systematic Reviews* 2006;(2):CD001292.

5 Lancaster T, Stead LF. Individual behavioural counselling for smoking cessation [online]. *Cochrane Database of Systematic Reviews* 2005;(2):CD001292.

6 Lancaster T, Stead LF. Group behaviour therapy programmes for smoking cessation. *Cochrane Database of Systematic Reviews* 2005;(2):CD001007.

7 Lancaster T, Stead LF. Self-help interventions for smoking cessation. *Cochrane Database of Systematic Reviews* 2005;(3):CD001118.

8 Lancaster T, Hajek P, Stead LF, West R, Jarvis MJ. Prevention of relapse after quitting smoking a systematic review of trials. *Archives of Internal Medicine* 2006;166:828–35.

9 Silagy C, Lancaster T, Stead L, Mant D, Fowler G. Nicotine replacement therapy for smoking cessation. *Cochrane Database of Systematic Reviews* 2004;(3):CD000146.

10 Stead LF, Perera R, Lancaster T. Telephone counselling for smoking cessation (Review). *Cochrane Database of Systematic Reviews* 2007;(3):CD002850.

11 Stead LF, Perera R, Bullen C. Nicotine replacement therapy for smoking cessation. *Cochrane Database of Systematic Reviews* 2008;(1):CD000146.

12 National Institute for Health and Clinical Excellence. *NICE Public Health Guidance 10: Smoking cessation services in primary care, pharmacies, local authorities and workplaces, particularly for manual working groups, pregnant women and hard to reach communities.* London: NICE, 2008.

13 National Institute of Clinical Excellence. *Brief interventions and referral for smoking cessation in primary care and other settings: NICE public health intervention guidance.* London: NICE, 2006.

14 McManus S, Meltzer H, Campion J. *Cigarette smoking and mental health in England.* Data from the Adult Psychiatric Morbidity Survey 2007. London: National Centre for Social Research, 2010.

15 Rigotti NA, Clair C, Munafo MR, Stead LF. Interventions for smoking cessation in hospitalised patients (Review). *Cochrane Database of Systematic Reviews* 2012;(5):CD001837.

16 Chong SA, Ong YY, Subramaniam M, *et al.* An assessment of the understanding and motivations of patients with schizophrenia about participating in a clinical trial. *Contemporary Clinical Trials* 2009;30:446–50.

17 Gierisch J, Bastian L, Calhoun P, McDuffie J, Williams J. Smoking cessation interventions for patients with depression: a systematic review and meta-analysis. *Journal of General Internal Medicine* 2012;27:351–60.

18 Lawn S. Systematic barriers to quitting smoking among institutionalised public mental health service populations: a comparison of two Australian sites. *International Journal of Social Psychiatry* 2004;39:866–85.

19 Lawn S, Pols R. Smoking bans in psychiatric in-patient settings? A review of the research. *Australian and New Zealand Journal of Psychiatry* 2005;39:855–66.

20 Lawn S, Condon J. Psychiatric nurses' ethical stance on cigarette smoking by patients: Determinants and dilemmas in their role in supporting cerssation. *International Journal of Mental Health* 2006;15(111):118.

21 Prochaska JJ. Smoking and mental illness: breaking the link. *New England Journal of Medicine* 2011;365:196–8.

22 Ratschen E, Britton J, McNeill A. The smoking culture in psychiatry: time for change. *British Journal of Psychiatry* 2011;198:6–7.

23 Williams JM, Ziedonis D. Addressing tobacco among individuals with a mental illness or an addiction. *Addictive Behaviour* 2004;29:1067–80.

24 Banham L, Gilbody S. Smoking cessation in severe mental illness: what works? *Addiction* 2010;105:1176–89.

25 Tsoi DT, Porwal M, Webster AC. Interventions for smoking cessation and reduction in individuals with schizophrenia. *Cochrane Database of Systematic Reviews* 2010;(6):CD007253.

26 Tsoi DT, Porwal M, Webster AC. Efficacy and safety of bupropion for smoking cessation and reduction in schizophrenia: systematic review and meta-analysis. *British Journal of Psychiatry* 2010;196:346.

27 Yousefi M, Folsom T, Fatemi H. A review of the efficacy and tolerability of varenicline in smoking cessation studies in subjects with schizophrenia. *Journal of Addiction Research and Therapy* 2011;S4:3045.

28 McEwen A, West R, McRobbie H. Effectiveness of specialist group treatment for smoking cessation vs. one-to-one treatment in primary care. *Addictive Behaviors* 2006;31:1650–60.

29 George TP, Ziedonis DM, Feingold A, *et al*. Nicotine transdermal patch and atypical antipsychotic medications for smoking cessation in schizophrenia. *American Journal of Psychiatry* 2000;157:1835–42.

30 Baker A, Richmond R, Haile M, *et al*. A randomized controlled trial of a smoking cessation intervention among people with a psychotic disorder. *American Journal of Psychiatry* 2006;163:1934–42.

31 Campion J, Hewitt J, Shiers D, Taylor D (2010) Pharmacy guidance on smoking and mental health. Forum for Mental Health in Primary Care. www.rcpsych.ac.uk/pdf/Pharmacy_%20guidance%20for%20smoking%20and%20mental%20health%20Feb%202010.pdf [Accessed 20 February 2013]

32 Weiser M, Reichenberg A, Grotto I. Higher rates of cigarette smoking in male adolescents before the onset of schizophrenia: a historical-prospective cohort study. *American Journal of Psychiatry* 2004;161:1219–23.

33 Williams JM, Ziedonis DM, Abanyie F. Increased nicotine and cotinine levels in smokers with schizophrenia and schizoaffective disorder is not a metabolic effect. *Schizophrenia Research* 2005;79:323–35.

34 Williams JM, Ziedonis DM, Foulds J. A case series of nicotine nasal spray in the treatment of tobacco dependence among patients with schizophrenia. *Hospital and Community Psychiatry* 2004;55:1064–6.

35 Evins A, Mays V, Rigotti N, *et al*. A pilot trial of bupropion added to cognitive behavioural therapy for smoking cessation in schizophrenia. *Nicotine and Tobacco Research* 2001;3:397–403.

36 Evins A, Cather C, Deckersbach T, *et al*. Double-blind, placebo-controlled trial of bupropion sustained-release for smoking cessation in schizophrenia. *Journal of Clinical Psychopharmacology* 2005;25:218–25.

37 George T, Vessicchio J, Termine A, *et al*. A Placebo controlled trial of bupropion for smoking cessation in schizophrenia. *Biological Psychiatry* 2002;52:53–61.

38 Evins A, Cather C, Culhane M, *et al*. A 12-week double-blind, placebo-controlled study of bupropion SR added to high-dose dual nicotine replacement therapy for smoking cessation or reduction in schizophrenia. *Journal of Clinical Psychopharmacology* 2007;27:380–6.

39 George T, Vessicchio J, Sacco K, *et al*. A placebo-controlled trial of bupropion combined with nicotine patch for smoking cessation in schizophrenia. *Biological Psychiatry* 2008;63:1092–6.

40 Gunnell D, Irvine D, Wise L, Davies C, Martin RM. Varenicline and suicidal behaviour: a cohort study based on data from the General Practice Research Database. *British Medical Journal* 2009;339:b3805.

41 Williams J, Anthenelli R, Morris C, *et al*. A randomised, double-blind, placebo-controlled study evaluating the safety and efficacy of varenicline for smoking cessation in patients with schizophrenia or schizoaffective disorder. *Journal of Clinical Psychiatry* 2012;73:654–60.

42 Pachas G, Cather C, Pratt S, et al. Varenicline for smoking cessation in schizophrenia: safety and effectiveness in a 12-week, open-label trial. *Journal of Dual Diagnosis* 2012;8:117–25.

43 Weiner E, Bucholz A, Coffay A, et al. Varenicline for smoking cessation in people with schizophrenia: a randomized double blind pilot study. *Schizophrenia Research* 2011;129:94–5.

44 Smith RC, Lindenmayer J, Davis JM, et al. Cognitive and antismoking effects of varenicline in patients with schizophrenia or schizoaffective disorder. *Schizophrenia Research* 2009;110:149–55.

45 Pfizer News and Media. New study with CHANTIX/CHAMPIX (varenicline) tablets suggests favourable benefit-risk profile in adult smokers with major depressive disorder, 2012. http://press.pfizer.com/press-release/new-study-chantixchampix-varenicline-tablets-suggests%C2%A0favorable-benefit-risk-profile-a [Accessed 20 February 2013]

46 MHRA. Stop Smoking Treatments. 2013. www.mhra.gov.uk/PrintPreview/DefaultSplashPP/CON2031590?ResultCount = 10&DynamicListQuery = &DynamicListSortBy = xCreationDate&DynamicListSortOrder = Desc&DynamicListTitle = &PageNumber = 1&Title = 'Stop%20smoking'%20treatments [Accessed 20 February 2013]

47 Food and Drug Administration. Information for Healthcare Professionals: Varenicline and Bupropion, 2009. www.fda.gov/Drugs/DrugSafety/PostmarketDrugSafetyInformationforPatientsandProviders/DrugSafetyInformationforHeathcareProfessionals/ucm169986.htm [Accessed 20 February 2013]

48 Pisinger C, Godtfredsen NS. Is there a health benefit of reduced tobacco consumption? A systematic review. *Nicotine and Tobacco Research* 2007;9:631–46.

49 Hughes JR, Carpenter MJ. Does smoking reduction increase future cessation and decrease disease risk? A qualitative review. *Nicotine and Tobacco Research* 2006;8:739–49.

50 Moore D, Aveyard P, Connock M, et al. Effectiveness and safety of nicotine replacement therapy assisted reduction to stop smoking: systematic review and meta-analysis. *British Medical Journal* 2009;338:b1024.

51 Wang D, Connock, Barton P, et al. 'Cut down to quit' with nicotine replacement therapies in smoking cessation: a systematic review of effectiveness and economic analysis. *Health Technol Assess* 2008;12:1–156.

52 Royal College of Physicians. *Harm reduction in nicotine addiction. Helping people who can't quit*. London: RCP, 2007.

53 National Institute for Clinical Excellence. *Tobacco – Harm Reduction*. Draft guidance. London: NICE 2012.

54 Dalack GW, Meador-Woodruff JH. Acute feasibility and safety of a smoking reduction strategy for smokers with schizophrenia. *Nicotine and Tobacco Research* 1999;1:53–7.

55 George TP, Ziedonis DM, Feingold A, et al. Nicotine transdermal patch and atypical antipsychotic medications for smoking cessation in schizophrenia. *American Journal of Psychiatry* 2000;157:1835–42.

56 Ratschen E, Britton J, Doody G, McNeill A. Smoke-free policy in acute mental health wards: avoiding the pitfalls. *General Hospital Psychiatry* 2009;31:131–6.

57 Meyer T, Lockwood G, Sujie X, et al. Neuropsychiatric events in varenicline and nicotine replacement patch users in the Military Health System. *Addiction* 2013;108:203–10.

58 McDermott M, Marteau T, Hollands G, Hankins M, Aveyard P. Change in anxiety following successful and unsuccessful attempts at smoking cessation: a cohort study. *British Journal of Psychiatry* 2013;202:62–7.

59 Lycett D, Murphy M, Aveyard P. Associations between weight change over 8 years and baseline body mass index in a cohort of continuing and quitting smokers. *Addiction* 2011;106:188–96.

60 Fontaine KR, Heo M, Harrigan EP, *et al.* Estimating the consequences of antipsychotic induced weight gain on health and mortality rate. *Psychiatry Research* 2001;101:277–88.

61 Zevin S, Benowitz NL. Drug Interactions with tobacco smoking: An update. *Clinical Pharmacokinetics* 1999;36:425–38.

62 Desai HD, Seabolt J, Jann MW. Smoking in patients receiving psychotropic medications: a pharmacokinetic perspective. *CNS Drugs* 2001;15:469–94.

63 Carrillo JA, Herraiz AG, Ramos SI, *et al.* Role of the smoking-induced cytochrome P450 (CYP)1A2 and polymorphic CYP2D6 in steady-state concentration of olanzapine. *Journal of Clinical Psychopharmacology* 2003;23(2):119–27.

64 Seppala NH, Leinonen EVJ, Lehtonen ML, Kari T. Clozapine serum concentrations are lower in smoking than in non-smoking schizophrenic patients. *Pharmacology and Toxicology* 1999;85:244–6.

65 Lowe EJ, Ackman ML. Impact of tobacco smoking cessation on stable clozapine or olanzapine treatment. *Annals of Pharmacotherapy* 2010;44:727–32.

66 Zullino DF, Delessert D, Eap CB, Preisig M, Baumann P. Tobacco and cannabis smoking cessation can lead to intoxication with clozapine or olanzapine. *International Clinical Psychopharmacology* 2002;17:141–3.

67 Derenne JL, Baldessarini RJ. Clozapine toxicity associated with smoking cessation: case report. *American Journal of Therapeutics* 2005;12:469–71.

68 Taylor D, Paton C, Kapur S. *The South London and Maudsley & Oxleas NHS Foundation Trust Prescribing Guidelines*, 11th edn. London: Informa Healthcare, 2012.

69 Benowitz NL, Peng M, Jacob P. Effects of cigarette smoking and carbon monoxide on chlorzoxazone and caffeine metabolism. *Clinical Pharmacology and Therapeutics* 2003;74:468–74.

70 Benowitz NL, Hall SM, Gunnard M. Persistent increase in caffeine concentrations in people who stop smoking. *British Medical Journal* 1989;298:1075–6.

71 Gandhi KK, Williams JM, Menza M, Galazyn M, Benowitz NL. Higher serum caffeine in smokers with schizophrenia compared to smoking controls. *Drug and Alcohol Dependence* 2010;110:151–5.

72 World Health Organization. *International Statistical Classification of Diseases and Related Health Problems* – 10th revision. Geneva: WHO, 1990.

73 Breslau N, Kilbey MM, Andreski P. Nicotine withdrawal symptoms and psychiatric disorders: findings from an epidemiologic study of young adults. *American Journal of Psychiatry* 1992;149:464–9.

74 Gray KM, Baker NL, Carpenter MJ, Lewis AL, Upadhyaya HP. Attention-Deficit/Hyperactivity Disorder confounds nicotine withdrawal self-report in adolescent smokers. *American Journal on Addictions* 2010;19:325–31.

75 Piper ME, Cook JW, Schlam TR, Jorenby DE, Baker TB. Anxiety diagnoses in smokers seeking cessation treatment: relations with tobacco dependence, withdrawal, outcome and response to treatment. *Addiction* 2011;106(:418–27.

76 Tidey JW, Rohsenow DJ, Kaplan GB, Swift RM, Adolfo AB. Effects of smoking abstinence, smoking cues and nicotine replacement in smokers with schizophrenia and controls. *Nicotine and Tobacco Research* 2008;10:1047–56.

77 Allen MH, Debanne M, Lazignac C, *et al.* Effect of nicotine replacement therapy on agitation in smokers with schizophrenia: A double-blind, randomized, placebo-controlled study. *American Journal of Psychiatry* 2011;168:395–9.

78 George TP, Sernyak MJ, Ziedonis DM, Woods SW. Effects of clozapine on smoking in chronic schizophrenic outpatients. *Journal of Clinical Psychiatry* 1995;56:344–6.

79 McEvoy J, Freudenreich O, Levin E, Rose J. Haloperidol increases smoking in patients with schizophrenia. *Psychopharmacology* 1995;119:124–6.

80 McEvoy J, Freudenreich O, McGee M, VanderZwaag C. Clozapine decreases smoking in patients with chronic schizophrenia. *Biological Psychiatry* 1995;37(8):550–2.

81 Adler LE, Olincy A, Cawthra EM, *et al*. Varied effects of atypical neuroleptics on P50 auditory gating in schizophrenia patients. *American Journal of Psychiatry* 2004;161:1822–8.

82 HM Government. *No health without mental health: a cross-governmental outcome strategy for people of all ages*. Guidance. London: HMSO, 2011.

83 British Medical Association, NHS Employers. *Quality and outcomes framework guidance for GMS contract 2011/12. Delivering investment in general practice*. London: The NHS Confederation (Employers) Co. Ltd, 2011.

84 Coleman T. ABC of smoking cessation. Use of simple advice and behavioural support. *British Medical Journal* 2004;328: 397–9.

85 Thorndike AN, Stafford RS, Rigotti NA. US physicians' treatment of smoking in outpatients with psychiatric diagnoses. *Nicotine and Tobacco Research* 2001;3:85–91.

86 Department of Health. *Service users and carers and the care programme approach. Making the service work for you*. London: DH Publications Orderline, 2007.

87 Keizer I, Eytan A. Variations in smoking during hospitalization in psychiatric in-patient units and smoking prevalence in patients and health-care staff. *International Journal of Social Psychiatry* 2005;51:317–28.

88 Ratschen E, Britton J, Doody G, McNeill A. Smoking attitudes, behaviour and nicotine dependence among among mental health acute inpatients:an exploratory study. *International Journal of Social Psychiatry* 2010;56:107–18.

89 Glasgow RE. Changes in smoking associated with hospitalization: Quit rates, predictive variables, and intervention implications. *American Journal of Health Promotion* 1991;6:24–9.

90 Siru R, Hulse GK, Khan RJK, Tait RJ. Motivation to quit smoking among hospitalised individuals with and without mental health disorders. *Australian and New Zealand Journal of Psychiatry* 2010;44:640–7.

91 Lawn SJ. Systemic barriers to quitting smoking among institutionalised public mental health service populations: a comparison of two Australian sites. *International Journal of Social Psychiatry* 2004;50:204–15.

92 Myles N, Newall HD, Curtis J, *et al*. Tobacco use before, at and after first-episode of psychosis – a systematic meta-analysis. *Journal of Clinical Psychiatry* 2011;73:468–75.

93 Department of Health. *Smoking kills: a white paper on tobacco*. London: HMSO, 1998.

94 NHS Information Centre. *Statistics on NHS Stop Smoking Services: April 2010–March 2011*. London: The Health and Social Care Information Centre, 2011.

95 McNally L, Ratschen E. The delivery of stop smoking support to people with mental health conditions: A survey of NHS Stop Smoking Services. *BMC Health Services Research* 2010;10:179.

96 McNally L, Todd C, Ratschen E. The prevalence of mental health problems among users of NHS Stop Smoking Services: The effects of a proactive screening procedure. *BMC Health Services Research* 2011;11(190):online.

97 Department of Health. *National Local Stop Smoking Services, Service Delivery and Monitoring Guidance 2011/12*. London: DH, 2011.

98 Godfrey C, Parrot S, Coleman S, Pound E. The cost-effectiveness of the English smoking treatment services: evidence from practice. *Addiction* 2011;100(suppl 2):70–83.

99 Low A, Unsworth L, Low A, Miller I. Avoiding the danger that stop smoking services may exacerbate health inequalities: building equity into performance assessment. *BMC Public Health* 2007;7(1):198.

100 McNally L. Quitting in mind;a guide to implementing stop smoking support in mental health settings. www.quittinginmind.net [Accessed 20 February 2013]

101 Parker C, McNeill A, Ratschen E. Tailored tobacco dependence support for mental health patients: A model for inpatient and community services. *Addiction* 2012;107(suppl 2):18–25.

6 Population strategies to prevent smoking in mental disorders

6.1 Introduction

The smoking cessation interventions outlined in Chapter 5 offer effective support for smokers who want to quit, but their success at an individual level, and indeed their uptake, depends on individual motivation. As in all smokers, motivation to quit varies substantially between and within smokers with mental disorders, and is influenced by a range of factors operating at the population as well as the individual level including, for example, health promotion campaigns in the media, the price of tobacco, local and national smoke-free policies, the prevalence of smoking among peers and friendship groups, and many others. Many of these factors also influence uptake of smoking. Measures that reduce smoking in general, and smoke-free policies in particular, also reduce passive exposure to smoke and to the role-modelling effects of smoking behaviour on others.

This chapter reviews the population-level tobacco control strategies that contribute to smoking prevention, first across the general UK population, and then, where possible, specifically in mental health populations. The chapter also explores some of the institutional cultural barriers to effective smoking prevention in these contexts.

6.2 General population strategies

6.2.1 Smoke-free legislation

Under legislation that came into force in Scotland in March 2006, in Wales and Northern Ireland in April 2007, and in England in July 2007, smoking is now prohibited in almost all enclosed and substantially enclosed work and public places in the UK. The primary rationale for this policy, as outlined in the consultation process for the English legislation,[1] was protection of employees and the general public from involuntary exposure to tobacco smoke, although it was also anticipated that comprehensive restrictions on smoking in public and work places would stimulate quit attempts and hence reduce overall smoking prevalence.

Smoke-free legislation has, throughout the UK, proved to be popular, to achieve high levels of compliance, to improve air quality and reduce passive smoke exposure, and to have a positive impact on health outcomes.[2–7] The legislation also stimulated quit attempts,[8] although the longer-term impact on wider smoking prevalence, if any, appears to have been modest.[9] The legislation also appears to have changed smoking behaviour, resulting in reductions in passive exposure in the home,[6] although tackling passive smoke exposure, particularly of children, in these settings remains a pressing challenge for policy makers. The Royal College of Physicians has previously called for more effective policies to promote smoke-free homes, vehicles and a more extensive range of public places.[6]

6.2.2 Mass media campaigns

International evidence suggests that mass media campaigns are an effective means of increasing smoking cessation and reducing smoking prevalence,[10–15] although evidence specific to the UK is limited to older studies.[16–19] In recent years the UK government has invested in anti-smoking mass media campaigns highlighting the health risks of smoking, the hazards of passive smoking, the addictive nature of smoking and a range of other health topics, promoting National Health Service (NHS) stop smoking services, and in 2012 the *Stoptober* mass quit campaign. Media campaigns have also been used by pharmaceutical companies to promote use of nicotine replacement therapy (NRT) to quit smoking, and there is some international evidence that such advertising can have a positive effect on NRT sales.[13,20,21] Data from the UK data indicate, however, that pharmaceutical company advertising has less impact on quit attempts than government-funded campaigns.[22]

6.2.3 Health warnings

Evidence from the UK and elsewhere demonstrates that health warnings on tobacco products raise awareness of the risks of smoking and support quit attempts.[23,24] Health warnings have been displayed on cigarette packs in the UK since 1971, but the implementation of the EU Tobacco Products Directive in 2002 has required all tobacco products to display a written health warning covering at least 30% of the front of the pack, and an additional warning covering at least 40% of the back of the pack.[25] Graphic pictorial health warnings are more effective than text warnings, however, and these were introduced in the UK in 2008.[26,27] The 2002 Tobacco Products Directive sets out other regulations for labelling cigarette packs and other tobacco products, including the provision of tar, nicotine and carbon monoxide yields, although the validity of the last measures, and their effectiveness in communication with consumers, has been widely questioned. These and other labelling regulations are likely to change as a result of a new Tobacco Products Directive now expected in early 2013.

6.2.4 Ending tobacco advertising, promotion and sponsorship

Tobacco industry advertising and sponsorship encourages non-smokers, particularly young people, to take up smoking, discourages current smokers from quitting and hence increases tobacco consumption.[28,29] Cigarette advertising on television was prohibited in the UK in 1965, and an EU Directive has prohibited all other UK television tobacco advertising since 1991.[30–33] The Tobacco Advertising and Promotion Act 2002 prohibited most remaining UK tobacco advertising[34] in stages, beginning with press, billboard and direct marketing in 2003, point-of-sale advertising in 2004 and tobacco company sponsorship from 2005, in accordance with the most recent EU Tobacco Advertising Directive (2003/33/EC).[35]

Remaining media for tobacco advertising include point-of-sale displays, which have been prohibited in large shops in England from April 2012 and in all other shops from 2015, with similar legislation likely to follow in Wales, Northern Ireland and Scotland. Tobacco imagery continues to be common in the media, however, particularly in films watched by children and young people,[36] and is a strong determinant of smoking uptake,[37,38] which remains unchecked. Tobacco packaging is also a means of promoting tobacco brands and related imagery, and in 2012 the UK government launched a consultation on mandatory standardised packaging for all tobacco products.

6.2.5 Price increases

Raising the price of tobacco through tax is probably the most effective means of reducing short-term tobacco consumption,[39] and probably also of reducing smoking-related inequalities in health.[40] Globally, on average, a 10% increase in tobacco price reduces consumption by 4%;[41] in the UK the figure may be as high as 5%.[42] People on low incomes who smoke, and young people who smoke, are particularly responsive to these effects.[41]

As a result of successive tax increases, to the extent that tax currently constitutes almost 80% of the sale price of cigarettes, UK cigarette prices are now among the highest in Europe.[39,43] However, these increases have not kept pace with increases in income, and cigarette affordability is now around 50% greater in the UK than in the 1960s.[44] The impact of price rises as a disincentive to smoking is further undermined by the fact that cigarettes are in fact available in many different brands with a range of prices, providing the opportunity to trade down to lower cost brands, the availability of 10 packs of cigarettes, the lower cost of hand-rolling tobacco and the availability of illicit tobacco.

6.2.6 Illicit tobacco

Illicit tobacco undermines tobacco control policy by reducing the price of cigarettes, thus increasing demand and contributing to tobacco-related health inequalities; the most disadvantaged people who smoke, among whom the prevalence of mental disorders is particularly high, are twice as likely to buy illicit tobacco as the most affluent.[44] It has been argued, particularly by the tobacco industry, that smuggling is driven by high taxes, although this is not invariably the case.[45]

In the late 1990s, an estimated 20–30% of the market for tobacco in the UK comprised illegally imported cigarettes.[46,47] Since 2000, HM Revenue and Customs has taken measures to reduce illicit supply in the UK, and the market share of illicit cigarettes is now estimated at around 10%; however, the market share of illicit hand-rolling tobacco remains extremely high, at about 46%.[48]

6.2.7 Minimum legal age for cigarette purchase

Laws restricting access to tobacco, if well enforced, can reduce use in young people.[49] In 2007 (2008 in Northern Ireland) the minimum legal age of purchase for tobacco products in the UK was raised from 16 to 18 years, and appears to have had an impact on smoking uptake in England, where smoking prevalence decreased more in 16–17 year olds between 2006 and 2009 after the increase in age of sale, than in older age groups.[50] Proxy purchasing remains a problem, however.

6.2.8 Smoking cessation services

At an individual level, UK tobacco control policy is targeted at offering people the best help to quit smoking. Around two-thirds of those who smoke in the UK report that they want to stop smoking, and over half have made a significant attempt to do so in the past 5 years.[51] However, as only 3–5% of unaided quit attempts are successful, providing people who smoke with the support needed to increase the likelihood of a successful quit attempt is a fundamental aspect of tobacco control.[52] As outlined in section 5.3, in the UK the NHS provides access to free, local stop smoking services (SSS) for all smokers who want to quit. SSS are offered predominantly in primary care, pharmacies and community settings, and are effective, with around 14% of users achieving validated long-term (12-month) abstinence.[53] The services are also highly cost-effective and may help to reduce socioeconomic inequalities in smoking prevalence.[2,54] The NHS also runs a stop smoking helpline, which offers advice and support, free of charge, to smokers who want to quit. The main limitation of NHS SSS is, however, their limited reach, because only 5% of quit attempts are made with the support of the

SSS.[55] Given that SSS are extremely cost-effective it is therefore important to improve the availability, awareness, access and uptake of SSS among smokers making a quit attempt, to maximise the chances of success.

6.2.9 Preventing smoking uptake through school-based interventions

Cigarette smoking is a behaviour that generally begins in adolescence, and particularly during the years spent in secondary education. In England, only 9% of 11 year olds have ever tried a cigarette, whereas, by age 15, 55% have done so and 15% are regular smokers.[56] Schools have therefore been a focus of efforts to influence smoking behaviour and prevent smoking uptake. However, most of the published evidence evaluating the effectiveness of such school-based interventions is from the USA, and it is not clear whether these findings are applicable to the UK, where the context of the health and education systems, and extent of tobacco control policy implementation, is different.[57,58]

The available evidence suggests, however, that school-based health promotion programmes to inform adolescents about the prevalence and health risks of smoking, and programmes to teach young people social and personal skills such as decision-making, stress that management and assertiveness have limited impact on smoking uptake.[57,58] Interventions to make adolescents aware of peer, family and media influences on their behaviour, correct their overestimates of smoking prevalence in their peers and society as a whole, and encourage them to make public commitments not to smoke, have been reported to have positive short-term and longer-term effects on youth smoking prevalence, but these findings have not been confirmed in higher-quality studies.[58] The UK ASSIST study has demonstrated that a peer-led education programme reduces uptake of smoking in young people in the short term,[59] although it is not clear whether this effect is sustained. It has been suggested that more comprehensive approaches, which tackle wider societal issues and involve intervention with students' families and the communities in which they live, may also be effective.[57,60,61]

6.2.10 Harm reduction

The potential importance of promoting nicotine substitution for people who smoke and otherwise cannot or do not want to quit smoking has been highlighted by the RCP as a potential means to decrease some of the harmful effects of smoking,[62] and to increase the likelihood of future quit attempts (see section 5.3). Harm reduction, ideally comprising complete substitution of smoked tobacco with an alternative source of nicotine, offers substantial potential to prevent smoking-related disease and provides an alternative for smokers obliged to comply with smoke-free regulation. Section 5.3 summarises harm reduction in the context of smoking cessation interventions, as will be promoted in forthcoming National Institute for Health and Clinical Excellence (NICE) guidance,[63] but harm reduction also offers potential at the population level by making alternative sources of nicotine, of which electronic cigarettes are an example, available to smokers as a retail alternative to tobacco for use independent of smoking cessation, medical services or any commitment to quit smoking. The UK Medicines and Healthcare products Regulatory Agency (MHRA) is currently considering regulatory approaches to enable harm reduction while ensuring that alternative nicotine products are safe, and is expected to announce its new policy in the spring 2013.

6.3 Population strategies and smoking prevention in mental health

Although it is likely that all of the above strategies influence smoking behaviour in mental health populations, evidence on the impact of tobacco control interventions is generally based on population-based surveys, which are able to explore attitudes, knowledge and behaviours in a range of sociodemographic groups but do not typically identify people with mental disorders. Direct evidence on the effects of population strategies in people with mental disorders is therefore scarce, although the fact that smoking prevalence has changed so little over recent decades in people with mental disorders (see Chapter 2) indicates a relative lack of effect. Finding and developing more effective ways to measure and monitor the impact of tobacco control interventions in populations with mental disorders are therefore an important priority. The measure for which the most evidence exists is the introduction of smoke-free policies in mental health treatment settings.

6.3.1 Smoke-free policies in mental health treatment settings

As outlined in section 6.2.1, smoking is now prohibited, with few and specific exemptions, in all enclosed and substantially enclosed work and public places in the UK. In advance of the introduction of the 2007 smoke-free legislation, a 2004 government White Paper, *Choosing Health*, strongly encouraged all NHS trusts to implement smoke-free policies by the end of 2006, thus setting an example for health promotion. Guidance was provided for the implementation of comprehensive policies which, as a 'gold standard', should include buildings and grounds.[64,65] However, during the development of the smoke-free legislation, a debate arose as to whether mental health trusts should be exempt from the law,[66–68] on the grounds of the high prevalence and levels of nicotine dependence among psychiatric patients, the complexities involved in the relationship between smoking and mental illness, and perceived practical difficulties anticipated in enforcing smoke-free treatment environments. It was also argued that imposing smoking bans on long-stay patients living on mental health trust premises, and those detained under the Mental Health Act, infringed human rights and rights of privacy. On the other hand, proponents of smoke-free policy argued that to exempt mental health settings from the law would worsen and, moreover, institutionalise existing health inequalities.

The outcome of the debate in England was not to grant exemptions for mental health settings but to allow an additional year, to July 2008, in which to prepare to comply with the legislation.[69] Northern Ireland adopted the same approach, but, in Scotland and Wales, mental health settings were exempted from smoke-free legislation.

A survey of all 72 English NHS mental health trusts in 2007 revealed that by that time all respondents (79%) had in fact implemented indoor smoke-free policies, although with variation as to the extent of inclusion of outdoor areas.[70] Almost all respondents reported perceived challenges specific to implementation of smoke-free legislation in mental health trusts, particularly in relation to safety risks (such as fires caused by covert smoking) and policy enforcement.[70] However, a review of 26 international studies found that concerns raised before implementation, eg smoke-free policy might lead to an increase in aggression or number of seclusions, discharge against medical advice or use of as-needed medication, generally proved unfounded when the policy was introduced.[71] Another review, of 22 international studies, concluded that smoke-free policies had no longstanding untoward effect on patients in terms of behavioural indicators of unrest or compliance,[72] although there are reports of complications arising from abrupt forced abstinence among highly nicotine-dependent patients[73] (see Chapter 5). It is now recognised that smoke-free policies in mental health settings, although in theory an opportunity to promote cessation at the point of hospitalisation, have to be complemented by comprehensive cessation or abstinence support for smokers if they are to be successful.[71,72] There is also evidence that complete and rigorously enforced smoke-free policies in psychiatric settings are easier to implement, and more effective, than approaches that are incomplete and leave room for interpretation,[71,74] eg facilitation of smoking breaks for patients, which require staff to escort smokers off and back on to the ward, are disruptive and can lead to an untoward fixation on regularly facilitated smoking breaks, which then come to take priority over other therapeutic activities.[75] There is also evidence that, after admission to treatment environments in which partial smoke-free policies are implemented, patients who smoke may alter their smoking behaviour.[76]

A study of 135 inpatients in England found that 14% increased their consumption of cigarettes, 23% decreased consumption and two patients relapsed to smoking during admission. Boredom and stress, and using smoking as a means to socialise, were the main reasons given for increased smoking.[76] Similar results have been reported in other studies, showing that people who are

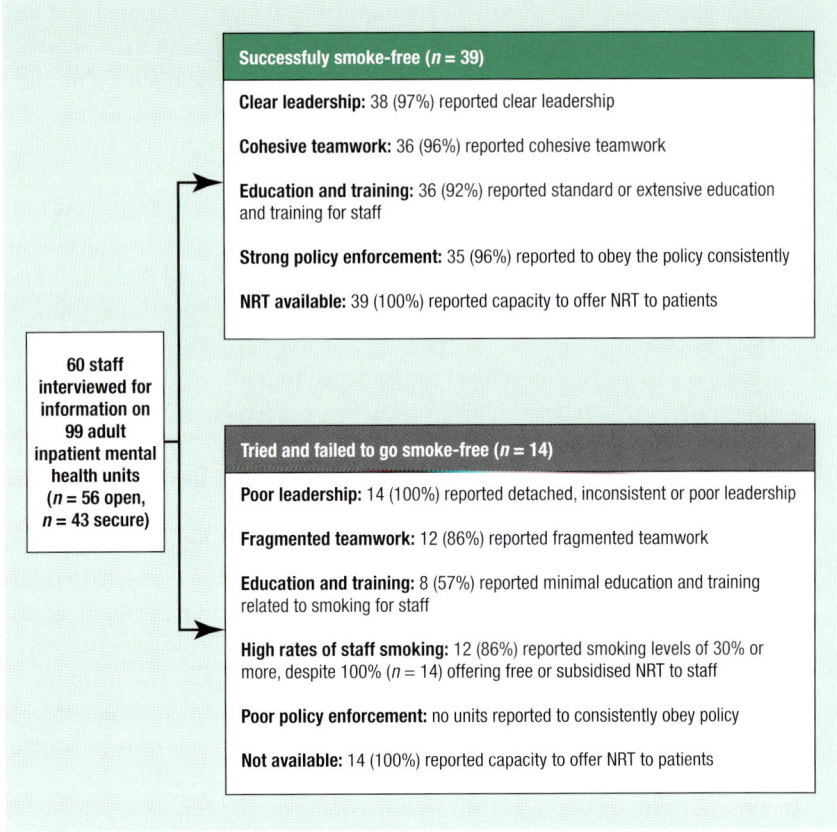

Fig 6.1 Determinants of successfully or unsuccessfully implemented smoke-free policies.[79] NRT, nicotine replacement therapy.

light and moderate smokers tend to increase, and those who are heavy smokers to decrease, cigarette consumption during admission to a smoke-free ward, consistent with an effect of imposed smoking pattern arising from restricted access to smoking areas.[77,78]

Figure 6.1 displays factors that have been identified as essential for the successful implementation of smoke-free policies across Australian mental health trusts, and include clear leadership, cohesive team work, consistent policy enforcement, staff training and appropriate use of nicotine replacement therapy (NRT).[79]

Studies of the clinical impact of smoke-free policies on symptom control among patients in smoke-free mental health settings suggest that there is no appreciable effect on the severity or improvement of symptoms in people who smoke relative to those who don't,[80] but can result in weight gain (an average of almost 5 kg in one study[81] – see Chapter 5, section 5.4.3). A systematic review on these effects, commissioned by NICE, is due to be published in 2013.

Follow-up studies of English mental health trusts 4 years after implementation of smoke-free policy suggest that the opportunity to use the policies as a driver of health promotion is being widely missed. Policy enforcement in mental health trusts is often deficient, with blanket exemptions being granted frequently to all smokers, and inadequate support from staff to address tobacco dependence among patients.[75,78] A recent assessment in a large mental health trust in England revealed that, despite a newly acquired focus on physical health,[82] addressing smoking was still a marginalised issue and not integrated into care pathways or standard procedures and documentation.[83]

6.3.2 Media campaigns

Evidence on the effect of mass media campaigns on smokers with mental illness is limited. One Australian study of 89 patients with schizophrenia[84] found that mass media campaigns did not appear to impact on smoking behaviour or intentions to quit in this group, and the authors suggested that tailored approaches taking into consideration specific barriers experienced to quitting may be more appropriate. The study also suggested that anti-smoking media campaigns may be less effective in marginalised populations in general, such as those of lower educational status and socioeconomic status, and those who are unemployed.[84] These findings are in line with suggestions indicating that public health campaigns to raise awareness of and prevent sudden infant death syndrome had less effect in people with mental disorders than in the general population, and implying that targeted approaches may be needed.[85]

6.3.3 Health warnings, advertising and sponsorship

We are not aware of any studies that have explored the effectiveness of health warnings, or relative impact of prohibition of advertising and sponsorship, in subpopulations of people with mental disorders.

6.3.4 Price and illicit supply

A US empirical modelling study suggests that mental disorders increase participation in the consumption of addictive goods but does not have substantive effects on price elasticity, and therefore that increasing the price of tobacco through tax is likely to be an effective means of influencing behaviour among mental health populations.[86] We are not aware of any British studies of this effect. Prevention of illicit supply of tobacco, which undermines tax measures, is likely to be effective because the most disadvantaged smokers, who are likely to include those with mental disorders, are twice as likely to buy illicit tobacco as the most affluent ones.[44]

6.3.5 Minimum legal age of purchase

Research exploring this issue with a special focus on young people with mental illness has to date not been conducted. However, as there is evidence that uptake of smoking occurs earlier among young people with emerging mental disorders compared with their peers without mental disorders,[87] this policy may be of particular relevance in mental health populations.

6.3.6 NHS stop smoking services

It is difficult to evaluate the impact of NHS SSS on smokers with mental disorders because relevant data on service use or effectiveness are not routinely collected (see section 5.3). However, based on the evidence outlined in section 5.1, there are no grounds to suspect that SSS are ineffective in mental health populations, although further research into models of service provision is urgently needed.

6.3.7 Harm reduction strategies

Harm reduction strategies for smokers with mental disorders, particularly serious mental illnesses (SMI), offer substantial potential for benefit. Given the typically high levels of tobacco dependence, the complexities involved in the association between smoking and mental illness (see Chapter 2), and resulting challenges in terms of motivation and confidence to undertake an abrupt quit attempt, often experienced by smokers in this group, offering harm reduction strategies could constitute an important step towards realising short-term gains such as reducing tobacco consumption (including its financial implications) and long-term gains such as increased likelihood to quit. Harm reduction could also contribute substantially to reducing tobacco-related health inequalities in one of the most vulnerable populations in society. To date, no research specifically exploring harm reduction strategies has been carried out, although a UK randomised controlled pilot trial involving tailored support including 'cutting-down-to-quit' strategies is currently being evaluated.

6.3.8 School-based interventions

We are not aware of any studies that have assessed the effectiveness of school-based interventions with a focus on issues around mental illness.

6.4 Factors perpetuating smoking in mental health settings

6.4.1 A smoking culture

Despite the scope of the problems caused or exacerbated by tobacco smoking in mental health settings, smoking among patients in these settings has typically been neglected, particularly by clinicians.[88,89] Consequently, although a societal change towards the 'de-normalisation' of smoking and prevention of passive smoke exposure in public and work places has occurred in the UK over recent years, smoking is still widely, if covertly, condoned in mental health settings. Indeed, the complexity of social and systemic aspects involved in the perpetuation of smoking in these settings is well recognised, and has been described as a 'culture of smoking', created and perpetuated by the coming together of 'various players, with various roles and rules for behaviour, interaction and communication, informed by beliefs and attitudes, set in the context of established rites, structures, artefacts and ideologies that together serve to perpetuate the culture'.[89] These conditions apply in relation to smoking in mental health settings.[90] Ethnographic and other work has demonstrated that smoking is a primary activity for mental health inpatients, forms a central part of the daily experience of both patients and staff, and has done so historically.[89] Smoking as a 'multifaceted tool' had become entrenched in the more complex set of social rules that apply in mental health settings and is used for purposes, such as the relief of boredom and stress associated with a ward environment, facilitating social interaction and the development of rapport between patients and staff, and controlling patient behaviour using cigarettes as a means of reward and punishment. Cigarettes have been described as the 'currency by which economic, social and political exchange took place', with patients and staff describing a complex enculturation process that involved strong reinforcement to smoke and rendered an escape from the culture in the studied settings extremely difficult.[89,91] Some important determinants that contribute to the perpetuation of the smoking culture are discussed in the following sections.

6.4.2 Staff beliefs and attitudes

The potential importance of the role of clinicians and other healthcare staff in promoting healthy behaviour in general and smoking cessation in particular is well recognised,[92] and staff beliefs and attitudes to smoking are important determinants and perpetuators of a smoking culture. The role of mental health nurses has been described to encompass that of a 'custodian, carer, cigarette source, counsellor, educator, behaviour modifier and gaoler'[91] and, although staff in mental health settings generally recognise the importance of health promotion for people with mental disorders, they also often report that they perceive smoking to be a personal right and expression of self-determination that they are not willing to question or undermine. There is also a widespread perception that smoking is of less immediate importance than other needs and priorities, particularly when patients are acutely unwell.[75,91]

Attitudinal differences between mental health staff according to smoking status and professional group have also been reported, with smokers being significantly more likely than non-smokers to believe that patients should be allowed to smoke with staff, to refer to smoking as a means of forming a therapeutic relationship, and less likely to think that patients who smoked should be encouraged to cut down or quit smoking.[93] In one British study, staff who smoked were found to be less concerned about the effects of smoking on staff and patients,[94] and nursing staff, irrespective of their smoking status, were less likely than psychiatrists to believe that patients should be encouraged to stop smoking, and more likely to think that smoking had value in terms of forming a therapeutic relationship.[94] Furthermore, independent of smoking status or professional group, staff believed that patients would become agitated or their mental health would deteriorate if they could not have cigarettes,[94] and a majority, including doctors, felt that smoking was an important coping mechanism that helped patients to deal with their mental illness.[95] Overall, smoking-related interventions are significantly less popular among mental health staff than among other healthcare professionals.[96]

6.4.3 Staff knowledge

Apart from attitudinal stances that may help or hinder engagement with smoking in mental health settings, it is also clear that knowledge relating to tobacco dependence and its specific links with mental illness, as well as behavioural support skills, are paramount to ensuring that smoking is addressed adequately. Such knowledge and skills are sometimes lacking. A survey of all clinical staff working in 25 adult mental health inpatient wards in England's largest mental health trust found that knowledge of tobacco dependence was limited across all staff groups including doctors, with clinically important facts, eg the need to monitor antipsychotic medication after smoking cessation, not widely known.[95] Misconceptions, such as the belief that nicotine constitutes the carcinogenic component in tobacco smoke, were also frequent (36%).[95] These findings indicate that the often limited support smokers receive on inpatient wards is further compromised by serious deficiencies in the knowledge of clinical staff, and therefore that appropriate training for staff on smoking interventions and culture is an important priority.[95]

6.4.4 Staff smoking

Tobacco smoking among nurses has been called both a 'contentious issue' and a 'conundrum'.[97] Contrary to expectation, smoking prevalence among nurses, who form the largest group of healthcare professionals and are viewed as public health role models, does not appear to be lower than that of the general population,[97] and in the case of psychiatric nurses may in fact be higher.[91] However, conclusive evidence on smoking prevalence among psychiatric nurses is not currently available.[98] British studies, some small, of smoking among mental health staff[93–95,99–102] report prevalence figures ranging from 17%[94] to 40%,[100] although the latter arises from a study conducted some 20 years ago when general population smoking rates were much higher. Similarly heterogeneous figures are found in other countries, often in the context of small sample sizes.[77,103–105] In line with general population surveys, some studies describe a gradient of smoking prevalence according to professional subgroup, with higher rates among non-qualified nurses (healthcare assistants) than in registered nurses, and lowest rates typically among doctors.[94,95,101] Despite the shortcomings of the available data, therefore,[97] it appears that smoking prevalence among mental health staff is broadly comparable to that in similar sociodemographic status groups.

6.4.5 Systems, targets and resources

Despite the growing recent emphasis on physical health in the context of treatment for mental illness, which includes prevention of premature deaths among those with mental illness and ensuring access to 'high-quality support services',[82] treatment of smoking is rarely integrated into care pathways. As discussed previously (see section 5.3), there is evidence that the structures and processes that would be required to ensure this[72] sometimes do not exist in mental health trusts, even if the smoke-free policy states otherwise. Recordings of patients' smoking status, or any other smoking-related information such as motivation to quit, support offered, referrals made or nicotine withdrawal experienced in inpatient settings, appear to be rare, although bespoke instruments to document smoking status and interventions, if available, are often not used.[83] The resources necessary to provide adequate support for smokers attempting to quit or abstain from smoking, such as a range of NRT products, behavioural support skills and staff time, are often missing. Overall, addressing smoking appears to occupy a very low priority in mental health settings[75,79,89] and, although this is in part a reflection of local factors, it also reflects inadequate national policy.

Apart from strategies discussed earlier (see Chapter 5, section 5.3), referring mainly to performance indicators, financial incentives and official guidelines to ensure that smoking is acknowledged as an important issue, overcoming prevailing misconceptions and negative or indifferent attitudes towards smoking by mental health staff is clearly an important challenge and priority. Efforts to integrate training and education on smoking and its specific links with mental illness into professional curricula, and to challenge the idea that smoking is a 'physical health issue', the treatment of which lies outside the remit and responsibility of mental healthcare, appear to be an urgent priority.

6.5 Summary

> - Population-level tobacco control policies have a significant effect on smoking prevalence in the general population by promoting quit attempts and discouraging smoking uptake.
> - Although specific evidence on the effect of existing population-level policies in people with mental disorders is lacking, the stability of smoking prevalence in mental health populations over recent decades in the UK suggests that they are less effective in this group.
> - It may be possible to increase the impact of some approaches, such as media campaigns, by tailoring to the specific needs of mental health populations.
> - However, it is also important to capitalise on the opportunities presented by contacts with mental health services to intervene to support smoking cessation and harm reduction.
> - Smoking is, however, a widely accepted component of the culture of many mental health settings, making cessation more difficult for smokers.
> - Smoke-free policies are a vital means of changing this culture.
> - Smoke-free policies are more likely to be successful and effective if they are comprehensive, and can be implemented successfully in mental health settings with appropriate leadership and support strategies for patients and staff.
> - Training and support to overcome prevailing misconceptions and negative or indifferent attitudes towards treating smoking among mental health staff are urgently needed.
> - Provision of effective smoking cessation and harm reduction support for people who smoke is crucial in maintaining smoke-free policy.
> - Investment in achieving smoke-free mental health settings, and in the support needed by patients and staff to allow this to happen, is therefore an urgent national priority.

References

1 Department of Health. *Smoke-free Premises and Vehicles: Consultation on proposed regulations to be made under powers in the Health Bill*. London: DH, 2006.
2 Bauld L, Judge K, Platt S. Assessing the impact of smoking cessation services on reducing health inequalities in England: observational study. *Tobacco Control* 2007;16:400–4.
3 Department of Health. *Smokefree England – one year on*. London: DH, 2008.
4 Holliday JC, Graham FM, Laurence ARM. Changes in child exposure to secondhand smoke after implementation of smoke-free legislation in Wales: a repeated cross-sectional study. *BMC Public Health* 2009;9:430.
5 Pell JP, Haw S, Cobbe E, *et al*. Smoke-free legislation and hospitalizations for acute coronary syndrome. *New England Journal of Medicine* 2008;359:482–91.
6 Royal College of Physicians. *Passive Smoking and Children: A report by the tobacco advisory group of the Royal College of Physicians*. London: Royal College of Physicians, 2010.

7 Sims M, Maxwell R, Bauld L, Gilmore A. Short term impact of smoke-free legislation in England: retrospective analysis of hospital admissions for myocardial infarction. *British Medical Journal* 2010;340:81.

8 Szatkowski L, Coleman T, McNeill A, Lewis S. The impact of the introduction of smoke-free legislation on prescribing of stop-smoking medications in England. *Addiction* 2011;106:1827–34.

9 Bajoga U, Lewis S, McNeill A, Szatkowski L. Does the introduction of comprehensive smoke-free legislation lead to a decrease in population smoking prevalence? *Addiction* 2011;106:1346–54.

10 Bala M, Strzeszynski L, Cahill K. Mass media interventions for smoking cessation in adults. *Cochrane Database of Systematic Reviews* 2008;(1):CD004704.

11 Durkin SJ, Biener L, Wakefield MA. Effects of different types of antismoking ads on reducing disparities in smoking cessation among socioeconomic groups. *American Journal of Public Health* 2009;99:2217–23.

12 Hyland A, Wakefield M, Higbee C, Szczypka G, Cummings KM. Anti-tobacco television advertising and indicators of smoking cessation in adults: a cohort study. *Health Education Research* 2006;21:348.

13 National Cancer Institute. *The Role of the Media in Promoting and Reducing Tobacco Use.* London: National Cancer Institute, 1998.

14 National Institute for Health and Clinical Excellence. *A Review of the Effectiveness of Mass Media Interventions which Both Encourage Quit Attempts and Reinforce Current and Recent Attempts to Quit Smoking.* London: NICE, 2007.

15 Wakefield MA, Durkin S, Spittal MJ, *et al.* Impact of tobacco control policies and mass media campaigns on monthly adult smoking prevalence. *American Journal of Public Health* 2008;98:1443–50.

16 Campion P, Owen L, McNeill A, McGuire C. Evaluation of a mass media campaign on smoking and pregnancy. *Addiction* 1994;89:1245–54.

17 McVey D, Stapleton J. Can anti-smoking television advertising affect smoking behaviour? Controlled trial of the Health Education Authority for England's anti-smoking TV campaign. *Tobacco Control* 2000;9:273–82.

18 Owen L. Impact of a telephone helpline for smokers who called during a mass media campaign. *Tobacco Control* 2000;9:148–54.

19 Sutton SR, Hallett R. Experimental evaluation of the BBC TV series 'So you want to stop smoking?'. *Addictive Behaviors* 1987;12:363–6.

20 Avery R, Kenkel D, Lillard DR, Mathios A. *Private Profits and Public Health: Does advertising smoking cessation products encourage smokers to quit*? Cambridge, MA: NBER, 2006.

21 Tauras JA, Chaloupka FJ, Emery S, *et al.* The impact of advertising on nicotine replacement therapy demand. *Social Science and Medicine* 2005;60:2351–8.

22 Langley TE, McNeill A, Lewis S, Szatkowski L, Quinn C. The impact of media campaigns on smoking cessation activity: A structural vector autoregression analysis. *Addiction* 2012;107:2043–50.

23 Hammond D, Fong GT, McNeill A, Borland R, Cummings KM. Effectiveness of cigarette warning labels in informing smokers about the risks of smoking: findings from the International Tobacco Control (ITC) Four Country Survey. *Tobacco Control* 2006;15:iii19–25.

24 Hammond D, Fong G, Borland R, *et al.* Text and graphic warnings on cigarette packages: Findings from the International Tobacco Control Four Country Study. *American Journal of Preventive Medicine* 2007;32:210–17.

25 European Parliament. European Parliament and Council Directive (EC) 2001/37/EC of 5 June 2001 on the approximation of the laws, regulations and administrative provisions of

the Member States concerning the manufacture, presentation and sale of tobacco products, 2001.

26 Fong GT, Hammond D, Hitchman SC. The impact of pictures on the effectiveness of tobacco warnings. *Bulletin of the World Health Organization* 2009;87:640–3.

27 World Health Organization. FCTC Article 11 *Tobacco Warning Labels: Evidence and recommendations from the ITC Project 2009.* Geneva: WHO, 2009.

28 Saffer H, Chaloupka FJ. The effect of tobacco advertising bans on tobacco consumption. *Journal of Health Economics* 2000;19:1117–37.

29 Smee C, Parsonage M, Anderson R, Duckworth S. *Effect of tobacco advertising on tobacco consumption: a discussion document reviewing the evidence.* London: Economic and Operational Research Division, DH, 1992.

30 The Television Act 1964. www.terramedia.co.uk/reference/law/UK_media_law/Television1964.htm [Accessed 1 February 2013]

31 Council Directive of 3 October 1989 89/552/EEC on the coordination of certain provisions laid down by law, regulation or administrative action in Member States concerning the pursuit of television broadcasting activities, 1989.

32 Directive 2001/37/EC of the European Parliament and of the Council of 5 June 2001 on the approximation of the laws, regulations and administrative provisions of the Member States concerning the manufacture, presentation and sale of tobacco products, 2001.

33 Directive 2007/65/EC of the European Parliament and of the Council of 11 December 2007 amending Council Directive 89/552/EEC on the coordination of certain provisions laid down by law, regulation or administrative action in Member States concerning the pursuit of television broadcasting activities, 2007.

34 House of Lords and House of Commons. *Tobacco Advertising and Promotion Bill.* London: The Stationery Office, 2002.

35 Directive 2003/33/EC of the European Parliament and of the Council of 26 May 2003 on the approximation of the laws, regulations and administrative provisions of the Member States relating to the advertising and sponsorship of tobacco products, 2003.

36 Lyons A, McNeill A, Chen Y, Britton J. Tobacco and tobacco branding in films most popular in the UK from 1989 to 2008. *Thorax* 2010;65:417–22.

37 US Department of Health and Human Services. *Preventing Tobacco Use Among Youth and Young Adults: A Report of the Surgeon General.* Washington DC: US Department of Health and Human Services, 2012.

38 World Health Organization. *Smoke-free movies: from evidence to action.* Geneva: WHO, 2009.

39 Mackay J, Eriksen M. *The Tobacco Atlas.* Geneva: World Health Organization, 2012.

40 Fayter D, Main C, Misso Keal. *Population Tobacco Control Interventions and Their Effects on Social Inequalities in Smoking.* York: Centre for Reviews and Dissemination, University of York, 2008.

41 Jha P, Chaloupka FJ. The economics of global tobacco control. *British Medical Journal* 2000;32:358–61.

42 Townsend J. Price and consumption of tobacco. *British Medical Bulletin* 1996;52:132–42.

43 European Commission. *Excise Duty Tables: Part III – Manufactured Tobacco.* Brussels: European Commission, 2010.

44 Action on Smoking and Health. *Beyond smoking kills: protecting children, reducing inequalities.* London: ASH, 2008. www.ash.org.uk/beyondsmokingkills [Accessed 20 February 2013]

45 Joossens L, Raw M. Cigarette smuggling in Europe: who really benefits? *Tobacco Control* 1998;7:66–71.

46 HM Revenue & Customs. *Tackling tobacco smuggling – building on our success. A renewed strategy for HM Revenue & Customs and the UK Border Agency*. HM Revenue & Customs, 2011.
47 House of Commons. HM Customs & Excise Annual Report 2000–2001. London: the Stationary Office, 2001.
48 HM Revenue & Customs. *Measuring Tax Gaps 2011*. London: HM Revenue & Customs, 2011.
49 DiFranza J. Restricted access to tobacco reduces smoking rates among youth. In: Owing J (ed.), *Focus on Smoking and Health Research*. Hauppage, NY: Nova Science, 2005: 77–100.
50 Fidler J, West R. Changes in smoking prevalence in 16–17-year-old versus older adults following a rise in legal age of sale: findings from an English population study. *Addiction* 2010;105:1984–8.
51 Lader D. *Smoking-related Behaviour and Attitudes, 2008/09*. Cardiff: Office for National Statistics, 2009.
52 Hughes JR, Keely J, Naud S. Shape of the relapse curve and long-term abstinence among untreated smoke. *Addiction* 2004;99:29–38.
53 Ferguson J, Bauld L, Chesterman JJK. The English smoking treatment services: one-year outcomes. *Addiction* 2005;100:59–69.
54 Godfrey C, Parrot S, Coleman S, Pound E. The cost-effectiveness of the English smoking treatment services: evidence from practice. *Addiction* 2011;100(suppl 2):70–83.
55 West R. *Smoking and smoking cessation in England 2010*. www.smokinginengland.info/Ref/Smoking%20and%20Smoking%20Cessation%20in%20England%202010%281%29.pdf [Accessed 20 February 2013]
56 Fuller E. *Drug Use, Smoking and Drinking among Young People in England in 2007*. London: The Health and Social Care Information Centre, 2008.
57 National Insitute for Health and Clinical Excellence. *School-based Interventions to Prevent the Uptake of Smoking among Children and Young People*. NICE public health guidance 23. London: NICE, 2010.
58 Thomas R, Perera R. School-based programmes for preventing smoking. *Cochrane Database of Systematic Reviews* 2006;(3):CD001293.
59 Campbell RSF, Holliday J, Audrey S, *et al*. An informal school-based peer-led intervention for smoking prevention in adolescence (ASSIST): a cluster randomised trial. *The Lancet* 2008;371:1595–602.
60 Carson KV, Brin MP, Labiszewski NA, *et al*. Community interventions for preventing smoking in young people. *Cochrane Database of Systematic Reviews* 2011;(7):CD001291.
61 Thomas RE, Baker P, Lorenzetti D. Family-based programmes for preventing smoking by children and adolescents. *Cochrane Database of Systematic Reviews* 2007;(1):CD004493.
62 Royal College of Physicians. *Harm Reduction in Nicotine Addiction. Helping people who can't quit*. A report by the Tobacco Advisory Group of the Royal College of Physicians. London: RCP, 2007.
63 National Insitute for Health and Clinical Excellence. *Tobacco – Harm Reduction: draft guidance consultation*. London: NICE; 2012.
64 Health Development Agency. *The Case for a Complete Smokefree NHS in England*. London: Health Development Agency, 2004.
65 McNeill A, Owen L. *Guidance for smokefree hospital trusts*. London: Health Development Agency, 2005.
66 Alam F. Exempting mental health units from smoke-free law. *British Medical Journal* 2007;333:551.

67 Campion J, McNeill A, Checinski K. Exempting mental health units from smoke-free laws. *British Medical Journal* 2006;333:407–8.
68 Julyan TE. Exempting mental health units from smoke-free law. *British Medical Journal* 2007;333:551.
69 House of Commons Health Committee. *Smoking in Public Places*. London: The Stationery Office, 2005.
70 Ratschen E, Britton J, McNeill A. Implementation of smokefree policies in mental health settings in England. *British Journal of Psychiatry* 2009;194:547–51.
71 Lawn S, Pols R. Smoking bans in psychiatric in-patient settings? A review of the research. *Australian and New Zealand Journal of Psychiatry* 2005;39:855–66.
72 El-Guebaly N, Cathcart J, Currie S, Brown D, Gloster S. Public health and therapeutic aspects of smoking bans in mental health and addiction settings. *Hospital and Community Psychiatry* 2002;53:1617–22.
73 Greeman M, McClellan TA. Negative effects of a smoking ban on an inpatient psychiatry service. *Hospital and Community Psychiatry* 1991;42:408–12.
74 Willemsen MC, Gorts CA, Van SP, Jonkers R, Hilberink SR. Exposure to environmental tobacco smoke (ETS) and determinants of support for complete smoking bans in psychiatric settings. *Tobacco Control* 2004;13:180–5.
75 Ratschen E, Britton J, Doody G, McNeill A. Smoke-free policy in acute mental health wards: avoiding the pitfalls. *General Hospital Psychiatry* 2009;31:131–6.
76 Smith J, O'Callaghan C. Exploration of in-patient attitudes towards smoking within a large mental health Trust. *Psychiatric Bulletin* 2008;32:166–9.
77 Keizer I, Eytan A. Variations in smoking during hospitalization in psychiatric in-patient units and smoking prevalence in patients and health-care staff. *International Journal of Social Psychiatry* 2005;51:317–28.
78 Ratschen E, Britton J, Doody G, McNeill A. Smoking attitudes, behaviour and nicotine dependence among among mental health acute inpatients:an exploratory study. *International Journal of Social Psychiatry* 2010;56:107–18.
79 Lawn S, Campion J. Factors associated with success of smoke-free intiatives in Australian psychiatric in-patient units. *Hospital and Community Psychiatry* 2010;61:300–5.
80 Smith CM, Pristach CA, Cartagena M. Obligatory cessation of smoking by psychiatric inpatients. *Psychiatric Services* 1999;50:91–4.
81 Harris GT, Parle D, Gagne J. Effects of a tobacco ban on long-term psychiatric patients. *Journal of Behavioural and Health Service Research* 2007;34:43–55.
82 HM Government. *No Health without Mental Health: A cross-government mental health outcomes strategy for people of all ages*. London: HMSO, 2011.
83 Parker C, McNeill A, Ratschen E. Tailored tobacco dependence support for mental health patients: A model for inpatient and community services. *Addiction* 2012;107(suppl 2):18–25.
84 Thornton LBA, Johnson MP, Kay-Lambkin F. Perceptions of anti-smoking public health campaigns among people with psychotic disorders. *Mental Health and Substance Use* 2011;4(2)110–15.
85 Webb R, Wicks S, Dalman C, et al. Influence of environmental factors in higher risk of sudden infant death syndrome linked with parental mental illness. *Archives of General Psychiatry* 2010;67:69–77.
86 Saffer HDD. *Mental Illness and the Demand for Alcohol, Cocaine and Cigarettes*. Cambridge: National Bureau of Economic Research, 2002.

87 Myles NNH, Curtis J, Nielssen O, Shiers D, Large M. Tobacco use before, at and after first-episode of psychosis – a systematic meta-analysis. *Journal of Clinical Psychiatry* 2011;73:468–75.
88 Glassman AH. Psychiatry and Cigarettes. *Archives of General Psychiatry* 1998;55:692–3.
89 Lawn S. Systematic barriers to quitting smoking among institutionalised public mental health service populations: a comparison of two Australian sites. *International Journal of Social Psychiatry* 2004;39:866–85.
90 Lawn S. *Systemic factors that perpetuate smoking among community and institutionalised public mental health service populations*. Australia: Department of Social Administration and Social Work, Faculty of Social Sciences, Flinders University, 2001.
91 Lawn S, Condon J. Psychiatric nurses' ethical stance on cigarette smoking by patients: Determinants and dilemmas in their role in supporting cerssation. *International Journal of Mental Health Nursing* 2006;15(111):118.
92 West R, McNeill A, Raw M. Smoking cessation guidelines for health professionals: an update. Thorax 2000;55:987–99.
93 Dickens GL, Stubbs JH, Haw CM. Smoking and mental health nurses: a survey of clinical staff in a psychiatric hospital. *Journal of Psychiatric and Mental Health Nursing* 2004;11:445–51.
94 Stubbs J, Haw C, Garner L. Survey of staff attitudes to smoking in a large psychiatric hospital. *The Psychiatrist* 2004;28:204–7.
95 Ratschen E, Britton J, Doody GA, Leonardi-Bee J, McNeill A. Tobacco dependence, treatment and smoke-free policies: a survey of mental health professionals' knowledge and attitudes. *General Hospital Psychiatry* 2009;31:576–82.
96 McNally L, Oyefeso A, Annan J, *et al.* A survey of staff attitudes to smoking-related policy and intervention in psychiatric and general health care settings. *Journal of Public Health* 2006;28:192–6.
97 Smith DR, Leggat PA. An international review of tobacco smoking research in the nursing profession. *Journal of Research in Nursing* 2007;12:165–81.
98 Rowe K, McLeod CJ. The incidence of smoking amongst nurses: a review of the literature. *Journal of Advanced Nursing* 2001;31:1046–53.
99 Bloor RN, Meeson L, Crome IB. The effects of a non-smoking policy on nursing staff smoking behaviour and attitudes in a psychiatric hospital. *Journal of Psychiatric and Mental Health Nursing* 2006;13:188–96.
100 Plant ML, Plant MA, Foster J. Alcohol, tobacco and illicit drug use amongst nurses: A Scottish study. *Drug and Alcohol Dependence* 1991;28:195–202.
101 Sainty M. Smoking and comprehension of the health risks. *British Journal of Occupational Therapy* 1985;48:8–10.
102 Tilley S. Alcohol, other drugs and tobacco use and anxiolytic effectiveness. A comparison of anxious patients and psychiatric nurses. *British Journal of Psychiatry* 1987;151:389–92.
103 Hay DR. Cigarette smoking by New Zealand doctors and nurses: results from the 1996 population census. *New Zealand Medical Journal* 1998;111:102–4.
104 Tong EK, Strouse R, Hall J, Kovac M, Schroeder SA. National survey of U.S. health professionals' smoking prevalence, cessation practices, and beliefs. *Nicotine and Tobacco Research* 2010;12:724–33.
105 Weinberger AH, Reutenauer EL, Vessicchio JC, George TP. Survey of clinician attitudes toward smoking cessation for psychiatric and substance abusing clients. *Journal of Addictive Diseases* 2008;27:55–63.

7 Smoking and mental disorders: special circumstances

The individual and population measures to prevent smoking uptake, and promote and support quitting, summarised in Chapters 5 and 6, are general approaches that apply across the spectrum of the population of people with mental disorder who smoke. This chapter addresses the special considerations relating to applying some of these measures, and particularly smoking cessation and smoke-free policy, in settings or populations that present particular challenges, or may require more tailored approaches. These comprise forensic psychiatric inpatient settings, prisons, people who misuse alcohol or other drugs, homeless individuals, pregnant women, and children and adolescents. Evidence is drawn primarily, but not exclusively, from UK sources.

7.1 Forensic psychiatric inpatient services

7.1.1 Introduction

Forensic psychiatric services provide psychiatric care to offenders with mental disorders, and to people with challenging behaviours that cannot be safely managed elsewhere. Patients are usually detained under mental health legislation or under a hospital order, with or without restriction, by the Ministry of Justice, or under legislation pertaining to other jurisdictions of the UK. About 4,000 people are detained in forensic services in the UK and, in a recent survey of forensic psychiatric service inpatients, over three-quarters had a diagnosed mental illness, with or without other mental disorders (the remainder being in the process of assessment for mental disorder);[1] over 50% of patients were transferred prisoners from local (remand) prisons, and over a third (36%) had committed crimes involving violence against the person.[1]

The aim of forensic psychiatric services is therapeutic and not punitive. However, security measures are necessary to manage risk and prevent escape; these vary from high to medium and low levels, and include physical structures, general policies and procedures, and relational security.[2] Healthcare staff are responsible for maintaining safety and security, and for delivering therapies to treat mental disorders and reduce the risk of reoffending.

7.1.2 Smoking prevalence in forensic psychiatric services

Reported smoking rates in forensic psychiatric services inpatients have been very high, at over 70% in one high-secure hospital,[3] and more than 80% in medium-secure settings[4,5] in England. As in other mental health settings, the high prevalence of smoking in forensic psychiatric services may reflect the patients' perceived need for self-medication, void filling and cultural pressure.[6] Patients in these settings may experience psychiatric symptoms, including those of mood disturbance and psychosis, and may use smoking to distract from or 'medicate' against such symptoms. Smoking can also be perceived as 'something to do' during prolonged periods of inactivity and boredom resulting from restrictions on movement and other security controls. Cultural aspects of the forensic psychiatric setting may also add value to smoking as a substitute currency, or if smoking is used to reward good behaviour or to facilitate engagement with patients[7] (see also Chapter 6).

7.1.3 Smoking cessation support within forensic psychiatric services

Guidance on stop smoking support programmes within mental healthcare settings recommends the routine delivery of brief interventions that feed into intensive, multi-sessional smoking cessation programmes delivered by suitably trained advisers.[6] In some respects, forensic psychiatric settings are particularly suitable for such interventions because long periods of admission provide time for patients to plan and implement smoking cessation, in close proximity to staff able to provide support throughout the quitting process. Smoke-free policies are crucially important to promoting cessation, as patients have reported high perceived levels of difficulty in stopping smoking when regularly exposed to other patients and staff smoking.[8] Overall the general points on smoking cessation provision for people with mental disorders, outlined in Chapter 5, also apply in this setting, although with the proviso that they must be compliant with security restrictions.

7.1.4 Smoke-free policies in forensic psychiatric services

In the UK, smoke-free legislation prohibited smoking in most enclosed public areas or workplaces in 2007, and in mental healthcare settings from 2008. In 2007, Rampton Hospital was the first high-secure hospital in the UK to become smoke free in buildings and grounds. Since then Ashworth and Broadmoor Hospitals in England and The State Hospital in Scotland have become completely smoke free. Some medium-secure services permit smoking in the grounds but not in the buildings, whereas others are totally smoke free.

Staff attitudes to smoke-free policies in mental health settings before smoke-free policy implementation have often been negative.[9] However, review level research evidence has shown that implementation of smoke-free policies in mental healthcare settings is unlikely to result in deteriorations in mental state, or increased levels of aggression, violence, use of seclusion, discharge against medical advice or increased use of medication on an 'as required' basis.[7] Nevertheless, consideration should be given to the relative advantages and disadvantages of implementation of smoke-free policies throughout all buildings and grounds, or limiting implementation to buildings and allowing smoking in all or selected outside areas (see Box 7.1 for examples). The successful smoke-free implementation strategy at Rampton Hospital was based on earlier experiences from mental health settings, and is summarised by Cormac and McNally.[10]

When the smoke-free policy was introduced at Rampton Hospital, 73% of the 298 patients were smokers. A survey before policy implementation showed that 76% of nurses believed that patients would be more aggressive if they could not smoke, 67% believed that self-harm would increase and 67% that patients would need more medication.[11] After the policy was introduced, there was an increase in untoward incidents in previous smokers at 3 months, but no increase in use of seclusion or psychotropic medication, and no fire alarms attributable to

Box 7.1 Some advantages and disadvantages of comprehensive and partial smoke-free policies

Comprehensive: buildings and grounds	Partial: buildings only
Lower security risks, as patients are not moving to other locations to smoke	Easier to enforce in settings with ready access to secure grounds
Simple to implement as smoke-free areas are defined by boundaries of the buildings or grounds	Problems may occur if access to outdoor areas is restricted
Less risk of passive exposure for patients and staff	Increased costs of providing extra staff to supervise outside smoking breaks
Patients have to quit smoking completely if they are unable to leave the forensic psychiatric services	Risks for staff if isolated with patients outside
Smoking breaks for staff during work time take longer, as staff have to leave the grounds	Staff may be exposed to tobacco smoke outside
Smoking by staff and visitors may be displaced to public areas and can cause nuisance	Risk of fires increased if patients retain tobacco and sources of ignition after smoking breaks
	Security risks from patients mingling in groups outside
	Patients are less likely to quit smoking, with continuing health risks

smoking. Nicotine replacement therapy (NRT; patches or lozenges) was widely used by patients, and in some cases for several months. In the 4 months after the policy was introduced, contraband tobacco and illicit ignition sources were found on seven occasions; there were no incidents of hostage taking or concerted indiscipline. Plasma levels of clozapine increased significantly after smoking cessation in previous smokers, necessitating increased monitoring and dose reductions.[12]

Key contributors to successful implementation included: high level management and clinician support; clear policies and strong leadership; financial resources for staff training, use of cessation medication, psychotropic medication monitoring, signage and additional staff complement at the time of implementation; staff training in cessation support; and prescribing cessation medications in advance of going smoke free. In 2009 the UK Supreme Court rejected a human rights legal challenge to the Rampton Hospital policy[13] (see also Chapter 9).

Other reported examples of success include Wathwood Hospital, a 56-bedded medium secure unit in England, where 90% of patients were smokers before implementation of a total smoke-free policy.[14] In the year after implementation there was no significant increase in rates of aggression or use of tranquillisers, and there was a reduction in conflict that previously had arisen over access to the smoking room. NRT was used by 54% of patients. Of these, 20% continued to use NRT a year after policy implementation. Four of twenty-three previous smokers treated with clozapine sustained a significant rise in plasma levels, necessitating dose reduction, after policy implementation.

At Mount Vernon Hospital in the USA, a total smoke-free policy was implemented in buildings and grounds in 1998. In a retrospective study of records from a sample of 140 of the 367 patients in the facility, there was a significant decline in disruptive behaviour and verbal aggression in moderate-to-heavy smokers, a 61% reduction in heavy smokers of 'sick calls' for physical complaints and, regardless of pre-ban smoking status, patients' body weight increased.[15] Use of NRT and bupropion medication was reported to be low (data not given). It was reported that staff and family members brought contraband tobacco into the hospital, necessitating periods of 'lock down' (full closure and movement restriction), and the use of more thorough search procedures.

7.1.5 Maintaining a smoke-free environment

Support from security staff is crucial in maintaining a smoke-free environment in forensic psychiatric settings.[16] During policy implementation, confrontation between patients and staff can be avoided by adopting a low-key approach to searches, by avoiding additional searches and giving patients various options for disposal of smoking materials. After the implementation, clinical and security staff should remain vigilant in case attempts are made to smuggle contraband smoking materials into the hospital. Carbon monoxide breath testing can be used to check whether a patient has recently been smoking. All new patients admitted to a smoke-free site must be informed that the hospital is smoke free and that smoking cessation support is available from ward staff trained in smoking cessation techniques. Management should ensure that sufficient staff are trained to support patients with smoking cessation, particularly on admission wards. Untoward incidents should be recorded and reported by staff according to standard protocols, and security incidents and violent incidents in forensic secure settings reported to the management, security department and clinical governance teams.

7.1.6 Summary points

> Smoke-free policies can be implemented successfully in secure forensic psychiatric settings.
> Key determinants of success include strong leadership, clear policies and communications, staff training and prescription of cessation pharmacotherapy in advance of implementation and afterwards.
> Well-managed smoke-free policies and adequate patient support can help to reduce risk to patients and staff in forensic psychiatric services.

7.2 Prisons

7.2.1 Introduction

There are 139 prisons in England and Wales, varying in capacity and security level from category A (highest) to category D (lowest) security risk. The category of prison to which offenders are allocated is determined by the crime committed, the likelihood of an attempt to escape and the attendant risk of harm to the public, and the length of the sentence remaining. Approximately 132,000 people pass through the prison system each year in England and Wales, with around 85,000 being held in prisons at any time. Some 95% of these are men, and most are under 30 years of age.[17]

Prisons exist to punish criminals, separate them from society, and correct and in due course rehabilitate them into the community.[18] Prisons also present challenges to health and wellbeing including: overcrowding, lack of purposeful activity and of mental and physical stimulation; fear, anxiety and mistrust; physical, emotional, sexual and financial exploitation; separation from family networks; and often inadequate medical care with an overemphasis on medication.[19–22] Prisons have entrenched cultures that shape the social relationships between prisoners, and between prisoners and staff.[21,23,24]

Although not primarily concerned with health, the prison service has a duty of care for those that it detains, which in relation to smoking includes promotion and support of cessation among smokers who want to quit, preventing uptake of smoking, and protecting prisoners, staff and visitors from passive smoke exposure. Doing so presents particular challenges, however, because smoking is an established and integral part of the culture and social norm of prisons.[25–27] There are also significant structural obstacles to the provision of cessation support to smokers, most of which apply to the general population of smokers in prison but perhaps especially to those with mental disorders.

7.2.2 Smoking and mental disorders in prison populations

Smoking and mental disorders are extremely common among prisoners and the wider population of offenders engaged in the criminal justice system. Recent estimates of smoking prevalence include figures in excess of 80% in both male and female prisoners[28–39] and in people on probation,[40] and probably at least 60% in detainees in police custody in London.[41] This is in part due to the extremely high prevalence, around 80%, of mental health problems ranging from schizophrenia and personality disorder to depression and insomnia, in prisoners (Box 7.2).[20,42] Prisoners and other offenders also have a high prevalence of substance and alcohol misuse, and low levels of literacy, numeracy and comprehension.[43] Over half of all prisoners and other offenders have no educational qualifications, and nearly half have experienced exclusion from school. They are also more likely to have experienced poverty and

> **Box 7.2 Mental health and behavioural characteristics of prisoners[20,43,46]**
>
> - 80% of prisoners have mental health problems
> - 72% of male and 70% of female sentenced prisoners have two or more mental disorders
> - 40% of male and 63% of female sentenced prisoners have a neurotic disorder
> - 7% of males and 14% of female sentenced prisoners have a psychotic disorder
> - 20% of male and 15% of female sentenced prisoners have previously been admitted to a mental hospital
> - 95% of young prisoners aged 15–21 have a mental disorder and 80% at least two
> - 20–30% of offenders have learning difficulties or learning disabilities that interfere with their ability to cope with the criminal justice system
> - Nearly two-thirds of sentenced male prisoners (63%) and two-fifths of female sentenced prisoners (39%) admit to hazardous drinking, which carries the risk of physical or mental harm. Of these, about half have a severe alcohol dependency
> - 77% of male and 82% of female prisoners smoke

unemployment, long-term disengagement from health and other services, and poor relationships with those who might help them.[44] Time in prison therefore presents a significant opportunity for smoking prevention and other health interventions among this otherwise hard-to-reach, disadvantaged and often otherwise neglected group.[45]

The motivation for prisoners to smoke is often linked to coping with the prison environment. Many prisoners smoke to relieve boredom or stress attributed to prison life,[26,47–49] but in practice smoking also arises from nicotine withdrawal, or because of peer-group pressure or the association with illegal drug use. Prisoners have reported feeling a stronger need to smoke while imprisoned,[3] while boredom, being confined to cells for long periods and stress have also been cited as reasons for relapse by prisoners who have made quit attempts while in prison.[50] As a male prisoner in an English category C prison remarked, tobacco is 'everybody's lifeline in here'.[21] Smoking habits also change in prison, both positively and negatively. The limited access to tobacco, in combination with other factors, may contribute to reductions in the amount of tobacco smoked and/or the frequency of smoking.[35,36] However, the high prevalence of smoking among other inmates can promote smoking, as, for example, in a US female prison in which 14% of prisoners started smoking for the first time and more than 50% increased their smoking after entering prison.[51]

7.2.3 Smoke-free policy in prisons

Smoke-free policies are intended primarily to protect prisoners and staff from passive smoke exposure, but, as in general society, also reduce the general acceptability and normality of smoking and hence support smoking prevention. Given the high prevalence of smoking among prisoners, passive smoke exposure in prisons can be extremely high; indeed, one study estimated that more prisoners in the USA die from exposure to second-hand smoke every year than from the death penalty.[52] As a result many countries, including most European Union member states, now impose restrictions on smoking in common areas in prisons, whereas in many parts of the USA smoking in prison is completely prohibited.[25,32] In New Zealand, all prisons became completely smoke free inside their secure perimeter on 1 July 2011, after a 12-month lead-in period and with free access to NRT for prisoners. Implementation is reported to have been successful, with no incidents of related violence, reported improvements in tensions between prisoners and staff, and with half of those who smoke stating that they intend to remain non-smokers after release.[53]

Smoke-free legislation was introduced in prisons in Scotland in 2005, and broadly similar measures in England and Wales and Northern Ireland in 2007; the Prison Service Instruction (PSI) 09/2007 for England requires all indoor areas of prisons to be smoke free with the exception of cells occupied solely by smokers aged 18 and over.[54] The Prison Officers Association has since called for more rigorous restrictions on health and safety grounds,[55] claiming that the PSI does not provide protection for officers when they enter cells. Establishments holding people aged under 18 years must have an entirely smoke-free environment within their buildings,[54] and most extend this to outside areas within the prison walls. Hence, Her Majesty's Young Offender Institutions (HMYOIs) which admit only juveniles, such as Wetherby, Hindley and Ashfield, are completely smoke free. In addition, one adult prison on the Isle of Man has been fully smoke free since opening in 2008.

7.2.4 Effectiveness and uptake of cessation services in prisons

Studies across a range of criminal justice settings in different countries have identified high levels of desire among offenders to quit smoking, and to receive support to do so.[9,28,34,37,39,56–58] Prisoners have described imprisonment as an opportunity to access smoking cessation support and NRT,[47] and qualitative findings demonstrate that many British prisoners want to 'achieve something' while in prison and view quitting smoking as a big achievement.[49] In an evaluation of NRT-based smoking cessation initiatives across 15 prisons in the north-west of England in 2004–5,[49] 41% of prisoners using the service quit for at least 4 weeks, comparable to quit rates in local disadvantaged populations at that time, whereas recent data on prisoners from the English NHS stop smoking services suggest a 4-week quit rate of around 55%.[59] These proportions are broadly similar to those achieved by NHS cessation services in general, as is the proportion of smokers using prison cessation services, at around 12% in 2010–11.[59] A recent pilot study exploring barriers and facilitators to the implementation of smoking cessation support across prisons in England[60] concluded that the prison service provides a generally favourable context for smoking cessation support and an important means of accessing hard-to-reach groups, but that the availability of a professional coordinator improved smoking cessation support in prisons and other criminal justice settings.

7.2.5 Design of prison cessation services

A range of smoking cessation delivery models, typically offering individual and/or group behavioural support, together with pharmacotherapy, have been used in criminal justice settings.[27,49,51,61–63] Although group therapy may be more effective in the general population of smokers, one-to-one services are sometimes required for reasons of security, and for prisoners who have difficulty coping with group dynamics. A study of 15 prisons in the north-west of England found that 9 offered both group and one-to-one support, 3 group support only and 3 one-to-one support only, all in conjunction with NRT.[49] In one British prison, 'rolling' groups were found to reduce waiting times for cessation support.[61] Prisons also differ over use of trained in-house prison service staff or specialists from community-based services to deliver support. In Scotland, smoking cessation is part of the work of the Enhanced Addictions Casework Service (EACS – equivalent of CARATS in England: Counselling: Assessment, Referral, Advice, Throughcare), undertaken by healthcare staff. There is no conclusive evidence on the relative effectiveness of these different approaches. Smoking cessation support materials for use in prisons need to take account of prevalent low levels of literacy, eg by the use of audiovisual materials.[61]

7.2.6 Regime issues

The movements of offenders within the criminal justice system can be a barrier to accessing smoking cessation services and to their success.[49,64] Transfers to other prisons are stressful and disrupt provision of behavioural support and pharmacotherapy.[49,50] Smoking cessation initiatives should therefore plan for the likelihood of transfers[50] by ensuring that medical records are transferred with prisoners, and a short supply of pharmacotherapy is provided to cover the interval until prescribing can be renewed at the new location.[49] It has been suggested that access to telephone counselling or quitlines may also help to overcome disruption to cessation service access associated with transfers.[26,64]

Release from prison can also obstruct the continuation of cessation support. As the post-release period is in any case a potentially challenging and stressful time of re-adjustment, relapse among those who have quit smoking while in prison may be particularly likely in this period. A US study of prisoners released from a tobacco-free correctional facility found that only 18% remained abstinent at the end of the first week after release.[65] Prison services may therefore need to link with community smoking cessation programmes to ensure support for prisoners after release.[26,61]

7.2.7 Staff attitudes and logistics

Negative staff attitudes to smoking cessation initiatives,[49] and a high prevalence of smoking among prison staff,[61] can be significant barriers to smoking cession in prison, as is the use of cigarettes, documented in a forensic psychiatry facility,[62] by staff as a reward or incentive to control behaviour. Engagement of prison staff in support of quit programmes, and promoting cessation among staff, is therefore important.[49,64] Delivery of smoking cessation initiatives in the criminal justice system can also place a substantial burden on prison staff who may be required to manage waiting lists, organise prescriptions and other paperwork, distribute nicotine patches and provide ad hoc support to quitters.[66] To be sustainable, cessation services in prison need to take account of these additional demands on resources.

7.2.8 Misuse of NRT

Cigarettes are often used by prisoners as a currency[26,67] and the same can apply to medicinal nicotine.[49,66,67] Prisoners have been reported to have accessed smoking cessation programmes to obtain NRT to sell to other prisoners, while continuing to smoke[66] or to steal or extort NRT from other prisoners. Some prisons have introduced exchange schemes, dispensing nicotine patches only in exchange for used patches, in response to this problem.[49] Some prisons insist on using transparent nicotine patches to prevent concealment of illicit substances. Most prisons prohibit all forms of chewing gum, including NRT; some prisons also prohibit foil wrapping or plastic containers.

7.2.9 Impact of mental disorders in the prison setting

The occurrence of mental disorders adds further challenges to the many institutional, logistic and cultural factors perpetuating smoking in prison settings outlined above. Prisoners with mental health problems may be victimised in prison society, and may experience difficulty engaging in cessation group work as a direct result of mental disorder, or because their vulnerability requires them to be moved at different times to the general prison population to avoid confrontation, and hence restricts access to cessation services. Concerns over the effect of quitting on ability to cope with the stresses of prison life may be a substantial deterrent to cessation, as are the problems of misattribution of nicotine withdrawal symptoms to mental disorder outlined in earlier chapters in relation to the general population of people with mental disorders. Monitoring antipsychotic medication blood levels as cigarette consumption declines may be more difficult in the prison setting, and historical concerns over potential adverse effects of varenicline and bupropion on mood have tended to inhibit the use of these treatments in prison settings. Collectively these various influences combine to perpetuate smoking among prisoners with mental disorders, and major changes are needed to reverse this effect.

7.2.10 Summary points

> - Smoking and mental disorders are extremely prevalent in the prison population.
> - Smoking is also prevalent among prison staff.
> - Smoking is heavily engrained in the culture of some prisons, and tobacco is also sometimes used as a surrogate currency.
> - Prisoners with mental health problems are likely to experience particular difficulty engaging with cessation services, and in quitting.

> However, prisoners are no less likely than the general population of smokers to want to quit smoking, and those taking up cessation support enjoy similar levels of success to the general population.
> As prisons, and wider society, have a duty of care for the health of those imprisoned, it is essential to challenge the smoking culture of prisons by making prisons smoke free, and cessation services widely available and accessible to prisoners and staff.
> Experience from New Zealand indicates that prisons can become smoke free without serious adverse effects, and that half of all smokers who quit as a result of imprisonment in a smoke-free facility leave prison intending to remain non-smokers.

7.3 Smoking and misuse of alcohol or other drugs

7.3.1 Prevalence of alcohol and drug misuse

In 2010 in England, 26% of men and 17% of women were regular users of alcohol at above recommended safe upper limits,[68] and in 2007 the Adult Psychiatric Morbidity Survey (AMPS) in England found that 8.7% of men and 3.3% of women are alcohol dependent.[69] For men, 7.8% showed mild dependence, 0.8% moderate dependence and 0.1% severe dependence. Among secondary school pupils aged 11–15 in 2010, 13% reported drinking alcohol in the week before interview.[68]

In 2001–12 in England and Wales 8.9% of adults aged 16–59 were reported to have used an illicit drug at least once in the past year, of which the majority had used cannabis.[70] Class A drugs (including opiates, cocaine, ecstasy and LSD) were used by 3% of adults,[70] and opiates and/or crack cocaine by just under 1%.[71] In 2011, 12% of 11–15 year olds used illegal drugs in the last year and 6% in the previous month.[68] Numerically these proportions translate into almost 3 million adults using an illicit drug in the previous year,[70] around 300,000 opiate or crack cocaine users[71] and about 1 million class A drug users. The prevalence of illicit drug use is highest in 16–24 year olds with 19.3% or 1.3 million using one or more illegal drugs, and 6.3% using class A drugs, in the last year.[70]

7.3.2 Smoking and alcohol or drug misuse

Smoking rates are particularly high among people with alcohol or drug dependence. About 46% of adults in England who are dependent on alcohol and 69% of those dependent on other drugs are smokers[69] and smoking rates in excess of 80% have been reported among those in treatment for alcohol or drug misuse, particularly in the USA.[72,73]

7.3.3 Mental disorders and alcohol or drug misuse

Mental disorders are associated with high rates of alcohol and drug misuse. Among 5–16 year olds in the UK, the most recent national child and adolescent psychiatry morbidity survey[74] reveals that drinking alcohol twice a week or more is 1.7 times more common among 5–16 year olds with emotional disorders, 4 times more common in those with conduct disorder and 2.3 times more common in those with hyperkinetic disorder. Cannabis use is 2.5 times more common among those with emotional disorders, 3.5 times more common in those with conduct disorder and 2.9 times more common in those with hyperkinetic disorder. Use of other drugs, such as opiates or crack cocaine, is 4 times more frequent in those with emotional disorders, 2.5 times more frequent in those with conduct disorder and 5 times more frequent among those with hyperkinetic disorder.

Alcohol misuse and dependence are also increased in adults with common mental disorders[75,76] and schizophrenia, with an estimated 43% prevalence of alcohol misuse in one study of first episode psychosis.[77] Rates of drug misuse are also higher in those with mental illness. Around half of those with a diagnosed severe mental illness such as schizophrenia or chronic depression abuse substances.[77–79] Among those in treatment for mental disorders in the UK, drug and alcohol misuse are estimated to occur in 20–37% of those in community mental health settings, 6–15% in addiction settings, and 38–50% in inpatient and crisis team settings.[80]

7.3.4 Impact of smoking in people with alcohol or drug misuse

Tobacco smoking is more hazardous to the health of people in treatment for substance misuse than their primary presenting substance of abuse. Of 222 deaths in a cohort of 845 individuals with substance misuse followed for 11 years in the USA, 51% were attributed to a tobacco-related cause of death, more than to alcohol or other drug use.[81] Furthermore, respiratory and other symptoms have been reported to be more common among smokers who abuse alcohol or opiates compared with non-smokers, although not in cocaine users.[82]

Tobacco smoking is also associated with a sevenfold higher likelihood of cannabis smoking,[83,84] and usually precedes cannabis use,[85,86] which in turn precedes use of cocaine and other drugs.[84] Among people with opiate addiction there is a direct and dose-related association between tobacco smoking and patients' subjective symptoms of inadequacy ('not holding') of methadone dose.[87] Smoking is associated with higher rates of illicit drug misuse in opiate treatment programmes[88] whereas reduced heroin use is associated with reduced tobacco use.[89]

The combination of heavy use of alcohol and tobacco multiplies the risks of upper respiratory and digestive tract cancers, including cancer of the mouth, throat, larynx and oesophagus.[72,90] Smoking also appears to impede the process of cognitive recovery after alcohol abstinence.[72] Smokers require higher doses of a number of benzodiazepines and opiates due to induction of liver enzymes by tobacco smoke (see Chapter 5).

7.3.5 Smoking cessation and alcohol or drug misuse

Contrary to popular perception, people in treatment for alcohol and drug misuse who smoke are often concerned about their smoking and interested in quitting.[73,91,92] Due to their two- to threefold higher rates of smoking and its impact on recovery, smokers with alcohol and drug misuse disproportionately benefit from appropriate smoking cessation service provision.[72,90] However, addressing smoking in the context of treatment for alcohol and drug misuse remains rare. A review of 342 drug misuse treatment units in the USA found that 69% offered no treatment for smoking cessation intervention[93] and, although equivalent recent data are not available for the UK, the historic negligence of smoking in the context of drug and alcohol misuse treatment is well recognised.[94,95] Commonly cited reasons for a failure to intervene in smoking include clinicians arguing the case of 'first things first', staff reservations over treating smoking and beliefs that cessation could jeopardise recovery efforts.[94]

However, the available evidence provides little if any support for these concerns, and if anything suggests that the opposite may be true.[72,90] Smoking cessation support can be integrated into treatment for alcohol and drug misuse without jeopardising recovery goals, and indeed can improve treatment outcomes, as discontinuance of one drug (nicotine) can support abstinence from other drugs due to shared neurobiological mechanisms.[90]

The evidence for effectiveness of smoking cessation interventions in those who misuse alcohol and other drugs is substantial. A meta-analysis of 19 randomised controlled trials of smoking cessation interventions for people in treatment for drug and alcohol misuse and in recovery showed that concurrent treatment of smoking resulted in a 25% increased likelihood of long-term abstinence from alcohol and illicit drugs.[96] This meta-analysis also showed that cessation interventions, including those that offered behavioural support but not NRT, were effective in patients with drug and alcohol misuse, doubling the likelihood of cessation during treatment for drug and alcohol misuse, and that interventions using NRT were more effective. Although these effects were not sustained in the longer term in the meta-analysis,[96] these findings and those of a separate review[90] provide clear evidence that cessation intervention achieves at least short-term benefit, and may enhance the success of other drug and alcohol misuse interventions. Results of a recent study employing intense tailored interventions,[97] with abstinence rates of 43% at completion, or one that integrated tobacco dependence treatment into substance abuse treatment pathways[98] indicate that further research exploring the effectiveness of bespoke interventions in this population is warranted in this group.[72,96]

7.3.6 Summary points

> Smoking is highly prevalent among people who misuse alcohol and other drugs.
> Smokers who misuse alcohol and/or other drugs are often concerned about their smoking, and willing to address it.
> Interventions to address smoking concurrently with alcohol and/or drug misuse are effective and can also support alcohol and drug abstinence. However, only a minority of those with alcohol and/or drug misuse receive smoking cessation interventions.
> Efforts to address this shortcoming through the development and assessment of more effective tailored treatment programmes, and through systematic integration into care pathways, are urgently required

7.4 Homeless people

7.4.1 The size of the UK homeless population

The number of homeless people, comprising those of no fixed abode who sleep rough or in hostels or night shelters, is difficult to measure. The Department of Health estimated that there were about 100,000 homeless people in England in 2007–8,[99] but this figure excluded the 'hidden homeless' such as those who do not use hostel services. The resulting underestimate is likely to be substantial, because a recent survey of 437 single homeless people found that 62% were 'hidden homeless' on the night that they were interviewed, and that the majority had never stayed in hostels.[100] The true figure may therefore be closer to the 380,000 estimated by the charity Crisis for 2003.[101]

7.4.2 Homelessness and mental disorders

Mental disorders, including substance abuse, are significantly more prevalent in homeless people than in the general population.[99] Homeless people in England in 2000 were more than ten times more likely to have psychosis, four times more likely to have a current common mental disorder and over five times more likely to be dependent on alcohol or other drugs.[102] A more recent review suggests that mental illness and alcohol or drug misuse occur together in around 10–20% of the homeless population,[103] whereas research from a London-based charity for homeless people found that around a third (32%) of service users were alcohol dependent, almost two-thirds (63%) had a drug dependency, 35% had a diagnosed severe mental disorder, and undiagnosed and untreated anxiety and depression were highly prevalent.[104] A study of homeless people aged 16–21 years revealed that over 60% met diagnostic criteria for post-traumatic stress disorder, and that over a third had made at least one suicide attempt at some point in their lives.[105] Other evidence suggests that mental disorders are strong determinants of homelessness, particularly for personality disorder, which may occur in up to 60% of the homeless population.[106]

7.4.3 Smoking and homelessness

The prevalence of smoking in the homeless population is also extremely high. A national audit of more than 700 homeless people in England identified an overall prevalence of 77%,[107] whereas an earlier UK study found smoking rates of 93% among homeless young people aged 16–19, and 96% in 20–24 year olds.[108] Homeless people who smoke also tend to smoke more cigarettes, to have started smoking at a younger age and to have smoked for longer than smokers in the general population.[109] Smokers among homeless people are more likely to be male, to have spent some of their childhood in care, to have dropped out of school, to be unemployed, to have been victimised, and to be dependent on alcohol or other drugs.[110,111] Similarly high smoking prevalence estimates have been reported among homeless people in the USA,[110–112] where the tobacco industry has marketed cigarettes specifically to homeless and seriously mentally ill individuals as susceptible and vulnerable consumer groups, and in this context has developed relationships with homeless shelters and advocacy groups.[113]

7.4.4 Excess mortality and health service use among homeless people

Homelessness is associated with substantially increased morbidity and mortality. Homeless people in the UK make around four times more use of acute hospital services than the general population, and eight times more use of inpatient health services than the equivalent general population.[99] The average age at death among those who remain homeless is 40–44 years.[99] This high morbidity and mortality are attributable to a spectrum of health problems including alcohol abuse, illicit drug use and mental illness; however, it includes a substantial component of diseases caused directly by smoking, including ischaemic heart disease, and lung and other cancers.[114] As for the general population, smoking in homeless people is the largest single cause of premature death. Ill-health in homeless people is further exacerbated by poor access to and uptake of health services; homeless people in the UK are 40 times less likely than the general population to be registered with a general practitioner.[99]

7.4.5 Smoking cessation in homeless people

In the context of complex life circumstances that often involve mental disorders, substance abuse and dependence, smoking and smoking cessation are often overlooked in the homeless population.[115] However, many homeless smokers are motivated and able to address their smoking. A cross-sectional study of 236 homeless adults in the USA found that 69% were current smokers, and 37% reported readiness to quit smoking within the next 6 months.[112] These individuals were more likely to have attempted to quit smoking in the past, and to have social support for their desire to quit. NRT was the most commonly preferred assistance method (44%). A trial in the USA enrolled 58 homeless people who smoked to a 12-week group counselling programme and cessation pharmacotherapy, and found that the average number of sessions attended was 7.2, most participants used at least one type of medication (67%) and 75% completed 12-week end-of-treatment surveys. Carbon monoxide-verified abstinence rates of 15.5% at 12 weeks and 13.6% at 24 weeks demonstrate that enrolling and retaining sheltered homeless people in a smoking cessation programme is feasible and effective.[116]

Although 55% of homeless smokers in the UK were recently found to have been offered smoking cessation advice,[107] data from the USA suggest that homeless people who smoke are less likely than the general population to succeed in quitting, with a lifetime quit rate of only 9%.[110] However, this would be consistent with the rate for other groups with high levels of tobacco consumption and dependence. Furthermore, as in mental health settings, homeless people who smoke report that the pervasiveness and social acceptance of tobacco use in homeless settings, together with perceived high levels of boredom and stress, make quitting particularly difficult.[117]

7.4.6 Increasing smoking cessation in homeless people

Helping more homeless people to quit smoking is important and requires radical change in the prevailing culture of smoking as the norm in hostels and other facilities for homeless people. Awareness of the immediate impact of smoking cessation in helping to reduce anxiety, stress, financial problems and antipsychotic medicine doses needs to be raised among homeless people and those who work with them, and flexible and innovative cessation services and interventions provided to meet their needs. Providers in emergency youth shelters are in a prime position to assess smoking, as well as substance use behaviours and associated risk factors; training and protocols for those working with homeless people should therefore address smoking and include guidance related to staff smoking, as smoking by staff is likely to undermine efforts to reduce smoking in this group. Encouraging service users to register with a GP is important to enable access to the full range of health services, including cessation pharmacotherapy and behavioural support through NHS stop smoking services.

The mental health strategy 'No health without mental health'[118] highlights a twin track approach involving early intervention for mental disorders, and promotion of wider population mental health. Acute mental health services have an important role to play in preventing homelessness by ensuring that people are not discharged from hospital with nowhere to go.[118] Coordinated smoking cessation provision, including relapse prevention, between primary and secondary care services is important to promote long-term cessation and early intervention if relapse occurs.

7.4.7 Summary points

> - Homelessness is associated with high rates of smoking and mental disorders, which contribute to significantly reduced life expectancy.
> - Homeless people who smoke are generally aware of the risks of smoking and the benefits of quitting.
> - Smoking cessation interventions are effective in this group, although, as is generally the case among heavily dependent smokers, success rates are relatively low. More intensive levels of support and high-dose NRT may be particularly important in this group.
> - To promote and support smoking cessation, it is also important to challenge the acceptance of smoking as a normal behaviour in homeless culture.
> - Staff working with homeless people need appropriate training to support smoking cessation and maintain smoke-free environments, in caring for the homeless.

7.5 Smoking, mental disorders and pregnancy

7.5.1 Smoking in pregnancy

Smoking is one of the main causes of birth complications, low birthweight, preterm birth and perinatal deaths, including stillbirths and sudden infant death syndrome (SIDS).[119,120] Adverse health impacts for the fetus exposed *in utero* are also known to extend into childhood,[120] and recent studies suggest that this may also apply to childhood conduct/externalising problems[121,122] and obesity.[122,123]

Women who smoke are more likely to stop smoking during pregnancy than at other times in their lives,[124] and up to 40% do so before their first antenatal visit.[125] However, cessation is much less likely among those who are still smoking when they begin antenatal care,[126] and in England in 2011 over 13% of women smoked throughout pregnancy.[127] Smoking through pregnancy is strongly associated with other markers of social disadvantage including low income, lower levels of education, domestic violence and mental disorders.[128–130]

7.5.2 Mental disorders and smoking in pregnancy

Mental disorders are common during pregnancy,[131,132] particularly depression,[133] with a prevalence of around 12%.[134] There is increasing evidence that women with mental disorders are at increased risk of poor pregnancy outcome, including low birthweight and prematurity,[133,135] stillbirth[136,137] and SIDS, and this is at least in part due to smoking. Mental disorders are strongly associated with cigarette use among pregnant women.[130,140] Current evidence is consistent with a self-medication hypothesis, whereby smoking is used to alleviate symptoms of depression,[141] but there have been few prospective studies of mental health in pregnancy in women who stop smoking compared with those who do not. However, there is evidence that smoking cessation in pregnancy is associated with improvements in symptoms of depression.[142] Public health campaigns, such as the SIDS reduction campaigns, also impact on antenatal smoking in women with severe mental disorders, although smoking rates in women with a history of a severe mental disorder remain high.[139]

7.5.3 Smoking cessation in pregnancy

Smoking cessation interventions in pregnancy are effective in preventing smoking and improving fetal outcomes,[119,124] although options for pharmacotherapy are limited by concerns over the safety of varenicline and bupropion, and uncertainty over the effectiveness of conventional-dose NRT.[143] Uptake of smoking cessation services during pregnancy is low, however,[144] and many women do not use NRT when it is prescribed.[143] The American Congress of Obstetricians and Gynecologists[145] and the UK National Institute for Health and Clinical Excellence (NICE)[119] emphasise that pregnant women who continue to smoke are often heavily addicted to nicotine and should be encouraged at every follow-up visit to seek help to stop smoking. However, translation of this guidance into practice is far from complete, and a recent audit in a south London hospital found that smoking was rarely discussed after the initial antenatal booking visit.[146]

7.5.4 Smoking cessation in pregnant women with mental disorders

Data from the UK suggest that primary care staff are less likely to record antenatal smoking behaviour in pregnant women with major mental health problems,[147] although recent UK data suggest that, when smoking is raised by health professionals, pregnant women with mental disorders are more likely to accept an offer of referral to smoking cessation services.[146] Similar to other smokers with mental disorder therefore[148] (see also Chapter 2), pregnant women are no less and may be more motivated to stop smoking, but are less likely to succeed.[146] Smoking cessation treatment outcome is also low among smokers with depression, particularly those with recurrent depressive disorders.[149–151] As discussed in earlier chapters (see Chapters 5 and 6), several authors allude to negative perceptions and attitudes of healthcare professionals as barriers to treating nicotine addiction together with mental health problems,[152] although there is limited specific research exploring this in pregnancy.

Smoking cessation interventions for pregnant women are thus in urgent need of research and development. One of few available studies, which comprises a randomised controlled trial of an integrated cognitive–behavioural therapy (CBT) intervention during pregnancy, addressing depression, partner violence, smoking and environmental tobacco smoke exposure in high-risk African–American women, reported that, although the intervention did not impact on smoking rates during pregnancy (possibly because there was a high spontaneous quit rate in the intervention and control arms), mothers in the CBT intervention arm were less likely to be smoking in the postpartum period and were more likely to reduce their environmental tobacco smoke exposure during pregnancy.[153] The intervention also significantly reduced the occurrence of very-low-birthweight and very pre-term birth.[154] These findings indicate that treatments could be particularly beneficial if integrated to address mental health problems in the context of problems such as domestic violence.[129] Tailoring of interventions to risk factors present in pregnant women who smoke seems important, because a randomised trial of an intensive depression-focused intervention for smoking cessation in pregnancy found that women with high levels of depressive symptoms receiving the depression-focused treatment achieved higher abstinence and improved depressive symptoms, whereas women with low levels of depressive symptoms had better outcomes if they received a control intervention.[155]

Although recent drivers such as the various NICE guidelines on perinatal care[119,133] have advocated routine screening by midwives for smoking, antenatal mental health problems and domestic violence, it appears that pregnant women with mental health problems need more support that is tailored to their needs. One strategy would be to target women with mental disorders before pregnancy by providing preconception counselling via mental health services;[156] this and other innovations to improve ascertainment, uptake and efficacy of cessation support are urgently needed.

7.5.5 Summary points

> - Smoking during pregnancy has significant adverse effects on fetal and child health.

> Women with mental disorders are more likely to smoke throughout pregnancy, but are also more likely to accept cessation support.
> Smoking cessation interventions are effective among pregnant women but may be more so if tailored to the specific needs and co-morbidities of women with mental disorders.
> Systematic and sustained intervention and support are necessary to maximise smoking cessation in this context.

7.6 Children and adolescents

7.6.1 Prenatal smoking and mental health in children and young people

Smoking in pregnancy has been linked to deficits in child growth and neural development including: effects on speech processing, irritability and hypertonicity in infants; behaviour problems in children; and modulation of the cortex and white matter structure and nicotine dependence in adolescents.[157] Prenatal exposure has also been linked to attention deficit hyperactivity disorder (ADHD) and other behavioural or 'externalising' disorders (see also Chapter 2). The prevalence of mental disorders is also higher among children whose mothers smoked during pregnancy, at around 25% in those whose mothers smoked over 10 cigarettes per day, 21% with fewer than 10 cigarettes per day and 14% in those with non-smoking mothers.[158] A longitudinal study of children at ages 5, 10 and 18 found that maternal smoking was linked with both behavioural and emotional disorders that persisted through childhood into adolescence.[159]

7.6.2 Passive smoking and mental health in children and young people

In 2007 around 22% of children in the UK, or about 4 million children, lived in homes where adults smoked regularly indoors, and this proportion was substantially higher in lower socioeconomic groups.[120] Recent cross-sectional studies in Scotland and the USA have demonstrated an association between second-hand smoke exposure, as measured by levels of cotinine, and poor mental health in children and young people. The US study of nearly 3,000 children and young people found that high serum cotinine levels in non-smokers were associated with symptoms of depressive disorder, generalised anxiety disorder, ADHD and conduct disorders, and that these associations were robust to adjustment for poverty, prenatal tobacco exposure, physical stress and other variables.[160] The Scottish study reported cross-sectional associations between passive smoking and mental health difficulty scores, and significant associations with hyperactivity and conduct disorder symptoms that were independent of socioeconomic status.[161] These findings are supported by a European cross-sectional study that reported an exposure–response relation between passive smoking and hyperactivity, inattention and conduct disorders.[162] Passive smoking in children has also been linked to neurocognitive testing deficits[163] and behavioural and emotional problems in general.[164]

7.6.3 Smoking and child and adolescent mental disorders

It is well recognised that smoking is particularly common among young people with mental disorders, especially emotional and behavioural disorders. Cross-sectional data indicate that, in Australia, 72% of young people with a conduct disorder had smoked within the past 30 days, as had 46% of those with depression and 38% of those with ADHD, compared with 21% of those with no mental health diagnosis.[165] In the 2004 Child and Adolescent Mental Health Survey of Great Britain, 19% of young people with an emotional disorder were classed as regular smokers, as were 15% of those with hyperkinetic disorder and 30% of those with conduct disorder, compared with around 6% in children without these disorders. Depression in adolescence has been associated with smoking in adulthood, whereas young people who smoke appear to be more likely to become depressed.[166] Adolescents with ADHD are more likely to smoke than their peers, to have started smoking younger[167] and to have more severe nicotine dependence.[168]

Theories underpinning the association with ADHD include nicotine self-medication, whereby young people smoke to alleviate ADHD symptoms by exploiting the central nervous stimulant effects of nicotine to improve attention and cognition.[168] This theory is supported by evidence that adolescents with ADHD who are not treated with stimulant medication are more likely to smoke,[169,170] and that children with greater levels of inattention and hyperactive–impulsive symptoms are more likely to be smokers.[169] Alternative hypotheses or potential confounders include the possibility that the impulsiveness, impaired inhibition and other cognitive deficits of adolescents with ADHD make it more difficult for them to resist initiating and continuing smoking,[168] or that the social disadvantages of ADHD result in greater exposure to peer smoking as a result of a higher likelihood of associating with deviant peers who are themselves more likely to smoke.[171]

Smoking is also more common among young people with eating disorders. The American National Longitudinal Study of Youth found that adolescent girls with a high body mass index, who reported that they were trying to lose weight, were more likely to initiate smoking than other females.[172] This association between smoking and dieting behaviours, and with disordered eating symptoms and some aspects of general weight concerns, may be more marked among females.[173] Similarly, although adolescents with anorexic-restrictive eating patterns did not use smoking as a weight control strategy, body image concerns were more prevalent in girls who smoked than in those who did not.[174]

7.6.4 Looked-after children and smoking

The prevalence of mental disorders among children who are taken into the care of their local authority is four to seven times higher than that of children living in private households.[175] The 2002 survey of the mental health of looked-after children indicated that these children have a high prevalence of risk-taking behaviours in general as well as increased rates of smoking,[176] finding that three times as many 11–15 year olds in care smoked as those living in private households.[177] Smoking rates in care are also high in Scotland, where 75% of young people in residential units reported smoking.[178]

As with the wider population of children, those in care who also have a mental health diagnosis are more likely to smoke. The 2002 survey data from England suggested that the prevalence among those with any mental disorder was around 50%, and among those with an emotional disorder 65%, compared with 19% of those without.[176] Emotional disorders and conduct disorders respectively almost quadrupled and trebled the chances of currently smoking in looked-after children (Table 7.1).[176]

Looked-after children living in residential care were also four times more likely to smoke than those in foster care, and those who had been in their current placement for less than a year were more than twice as likely to smoke as children and young people who had been in placements for longer.[176] However, according to one survey, over half would like help to stop smoking.[179]

There appear to be many factors influencing the high proportion of smokers among looked-after children. Interestingly, a survey of young people in residential units in Scotland found that only 27% had started to smoke while in care, indicating that many were already smoking when they left their birth families.[178] This is likely to be a reflection of the stressful or chaotic circumstances that may have led to being taken into care in the first place. The factors that affect smoking initiation in other young people, such as peers or carers smoking, may also have an even greater importance in looked-after children due to their vulnerability and need to build relationships. This is of significance, as one 2007 Scottish study[180] reported that a higher than average proportion of residential unit staff (two of five) smoked, and that almost a third were smoking in front of children and young people in contravention of

Table 7.1 Smoking status of looked-after young people aged 11–17 by mental health diagnosis (2002)[176]

	Emotional disorder (%)	Conduct disorder (%)	Any mental disorder (%)	No mental disorder (%)
Current smoker	65	51	51	19
Never smoker	20	21	23	45

guidelines. Young people in this study also reported that staff in residential care did not always take incidents of smoking seriously. Up to two-thirds of foster carers reported smoking in front of the children in their care, indicating that passive smoke exposure is also a significant risk for looked-after children. Other potential contributors include the reported low expectations of children in care,[181] particularly concerning education but perhaps extending to smoking as well. In crisis situations, and where placement moves are frequent, health matters may also take a lower priority.[182] Young people may miss out on health promotion messages and healthy lifestyle discussion due to school changes, or even due to being excluded from school.[183] These vulnerable children and young people, in terms of their mental health and smoking behaviour, are thus subject to a 'double disadvantage'. They have already experienced considerable adversity before coming into care and can be further disadvantaged by the care system itself. *Time for change*, the 2007 White Paper, with the key theme being the importance of good corporate parenting, states that 'the aspiration that the state has for these children should be no less than each parent would have for their own child'.[184]

7.6.5 Smoking prevention and cessation in children and adolescents with mental disorders and in looked-after children

In addition to the wider efforts to prevent smoking uptake in young people generally, there is a clear need for services to address the high rates of smoking in these groups. The Royal College of Psychiatrists recommends 'targeted approaches for children and adolescents with emotional and behavioural disorder, who are at a much higher risk of taking up smoking'.[185] This may take place within child and adolescent mental health services (CAMHS), but means that staff working with young people with mental health problems need appropriate training and resources to offer brief intervention or signposting.[186] British studies are lacking, but one US study of child and adolescent psychiatrists found that the majority did not give consistent messages about smoking, and highlighted the need for more formal training.[187] Some mental health problems may be open to specific approaches, eg it has been suggested that 'pharmacological treatment of ADHD before children are exposed to cigarettes may protect against smoking'.[171] NICE has produced guidance on smoking cessation services in general[186] and is due to publish guidance in 2013 on smoking cessation in secondary care mental health services; however, further research into what works is still needed.

There have been efforts to address the mental health needs of looked-after children through dedicated CAMHS teams and mental health screening. Similarly, there has been a movement to target smoking in this group in particular, eg by employing a looked-after children's smoking cessation adviser to work with young people, foster carers, social workers and residential staff.[188] In

Glasgow, a specific looked-after children's smoking cessation project was set up, involving health promotion advice, one-to-one support, and training of care staff around raising awareness and the importance of positive role models.[179] Given the association between smoking and mental illness, there is also a case for further integration and coordination of services, eg offering training on smoking cessation interventions to staff working in looked-after children CAMHS teams. Further work in these areas is clearly necessary.

7.6.6 Summary points

> - Smoking prevalence is high among children with mental disorders, and both smoking and mental disorders are common in looked-after children.
> - Professionals working with or caring for young people should provide positive (ie non-smoking) role models and be trained to deliver cessation advice and provide or arrange further support for those who want help to quit.
> - CAMHS should ascertain smoking status and provide cessation support as a routine component of their service.
> - In settings where young people are most vulnerable, such as adolescent inpatient units, there should be a broad programme of health promotion aimed at preventing initiation of smoking as well as smoking cessation.
> - Local authority foster care and smoking policies should explicitly protect children from passive smoke, and promote smoke-free foster homes.

7.7 Special circumstances summary

> - Smoking, and particularly high levels of nicotine dependence, are especially common among people in forensic psychiatric settings, prisons, homeless people, and those with alcohol or other drug misuse.
> - Smoking is also engrained in the culture of many of the institutions that care or provide for these groups.
> - People in these populations are no less likely to want to quit smoking, although the likelihood of success in any quit attempt may be lower than for the general population of smokers, and smokers may also encounter obstacles to engagement with existing cessation services.
> - It is therefore a priority to establish smoke-free cultures and to provide suitable smoking cessation support for all smokers, particularly those with high levels of dependence, in these settings.
> - Interventions to address smoking concurrently with alcohol and/or drug misuse are effective and can also support alcohol and drug abstinence.
> - Women with mental disorders are more likely to smoke throughout pregnancy, but are also more likely to accept cessation support.

> Smoking cessation interventions are effective among pregnant women but may be more so if tailored to the specific needs and co-morbidities of women with mental disorders.
> Systematic and sustained intervention and support are necessary to maximise smoking cessation among pregnant women.
> Child and adolescent mental health services, and local authority foster care and smoking policies, should explicitly protect children from passive smoke, and promote smoke-free foster homes.
> Professionals working with or caring for young people should provide positive (ie non-smoking) role models and be trained to deliver cessation advice and provide or arrange further support for those who want help to quit.
> In settings where young people are most vulnerable, such as adolescent inpatient units, there should be a broad programme of health promotion aimed at preventing initiation of smoking as well as smoking cessation.
> In view of the current lack of evidence on safe, feasible and effective tobacco dependence treatment in the settings and populations covered in this chapter, further research is urgently required.

References

1 Rutherford M, Duggan S. *Forensic mental health services: Facts and figures on current provision.* London: The Sainsbury Centre for Mental Health, 2007.
2 Kennedy HG. Therapeutic uses of security: mapping forensic mental health services by stratifying risk. *Advances in Psychiatric Treatment* 2002;8:433–43.
3 Cormac I, Ferriter M, Benning R, Saul C. Physical health and health risk factors in a population of long-stay psychiatric patients. *The Psychiatrist* 2005;29:18–20.
4 Meiklejohn C, Sanders K, Butler S. Physical health in medium secure services. *Nursing Standard* 2003;17:33–7.
5 Shetty A, Alex R, Bloye D. The experience of a smoke-free policy in a medium secure hospital. *The Psychiatrist on line* 2010;34:287–9.
6 McNally L. Quitting in mind: a guide to implementing stop smoking support in mental health settings. www.londondevelopmentcentre.org/mental-wellbeing/mental-health-and-well-being/smoking-cessation/quitting-in-mind-online-resource.aspx, source: NHS London Development Centre [Accessed 26 February 2013]
7 Lawn S, Pols R. Smoking bans in psychiatric in-patient settings? A review of the research. *Australian and New Zealand Journal of Psychiatry* 2005;39:855–66.
8 Dickens G, Stubbs J, Popham R, Haw C. Smoking in a forensic psychiatric service: A survey of inpatients' views. *Journal of Psychiatric and Mental Health nursing* 2005;12:672–8.
9 McNally L, Oyefeso A, Annan J, et al. A survey of staff attitudes to smoking related policy and intervention in psychiatric and general health care settings. *Journal of Psychiatric and Mental Health Nursing* 2006;12:672–8.
10 Cormac I, McNally L. How to implement a smoke-free policy. *Advances in Psychiatric Treatment* 2008;14:198–207.
11 Cormac I, Creasey S, McNeill A, et al. Impact of a total smoking ban in a high secure hospital. *The Psychiatrist* 2010;34:413–417.

12 Cormac I, Brown A, Creasey S, Ferriter M, Huckstep B. A retrospective evaluation of the impact of total smoking cessation on psychiatric inpatients taking clozapine. *Acta Psychiatrica Scandinavica* 2010;121:393–397.

13 N, R (on the application of) v Secretary of State for Health EWCA Civ 795 (24 July 2009). England and Wales Court of Appeal (Civil Division) Decisions, 2009. www.bailii.org/ew/cases/EWCA/Civ/2009/795.html [Accessed 26 February 2013]

14 Shetty A, Alex R, Bloye D. The experience of a smoke-free policy in a medium secure hospital. *The Psychiatrist* 2010;34:287–289.

15 Hempel AG, Kownacki R, Malin DH, *et al*. Effect of a total smoking ban in a maximum security psychiatric hospital. *Behavioral Science and the Law* 2002;20:507–22.

16 Moss TG, Weinberger AH, Vessicchio JC, *et al*. A tobacco reconceptualization in psychiatry (TRIP): Towards the development of tobacco free psychiatric facilities. *American Journal on Addictions* 2011;19:293–331.

17 Ministry of Justice. Prison Population Projections 2011–2017 England and Wales, 2011.

18 Watson R, Stimpson A, Hostick T. Prison health care: a review of the literature. *International Journal of Nursing Studies* 2004;41:119–28.

19 Birmingham L, Wilson S, Adshead G. Prison medicine: ethics and equivalence. *British Journal of Psychiatry* 2006;188:4–6.

20 Scott D, Codd H. *Controversial Issues in Prisons*. Berkshire: Open University Press, 2010.

21 de Viggiani N. Unhealthy prisons: exploring structural determinants of prison health. *Socioology of Health and Illness* 2007;29:115–35.

22 Howard League for Penal Reform. Prisons are Incapacitated by Overcrowding (press release 11 March 2005).

23 Sykes. *The Society of Captives: A study of a maximum security prison*. Princeton, NJ: Princeton University Press, 1958.

24 Liebling A. Doing research in prison: Breaking the silence? *Theoretical Criminology* 1999;3:147–173.

25 Butler T, Richmond R, Belcher J, Wilhelm K, Wodak A. Should smoking be banned in prisons? *Tobacco Control* 2007;16:291–3.

26 Richmond R, Butler T, Wilhelm K, *et al*. Tobacco in prisons: a focus group study. *Tobacco Control* 2009;18:176–82.

27 Long CG, Jones K. Issues in running smoking cessation groups with forensic psychiatric inpatients:Results of a pilot study and lessons learnt. *British Journal of Forensic Practice* 2005;7:22–8.

28 Belcher JM, Butler T, Richmond RL, Wodak AD, Wilhelm K. Smoking and its correlates in an Australian prisoner population. *Drug and Alcohol Review* 2006;25:343–8.

29 Cropsey KL, Crews KM, Silbermen SL. Relationship between smoking and oral health in a prison population. *Journal of Correctional Healthcare* 2005;12:240–8.

30 Cropsey KL, Eldridge G, Weaver MF, Villabolos GC, Stitzer ML. Expired carbon monoxide levels in self-reported smokers and non-smokers in prison. *Nicotine and Tobacco Research* 2005;8:653–9.

31 Cropsey KL, Jones-Whaley S, Jackson DO, Hale GL. Smoking characteristics of community corrections clients. *Nicotine and Tobacco Research* 2010;12:53–58.

32 Hartwig C, Stover H, Weilandt C. Report on tobacco smoking in prison: Final Report Work Package 7. Directorate General for Health and Consumer Affairs (DG SANCO). DG SANCO/2006/C4/02; 2008.

33 Holmwood C, Marriott M, Humeniuk R. Substance use patterns in newly admitted male and female South Australian prisoners using the WHO-ASSIST (Alcohol, Smoking and

substance involvement Screening Test). *International Journal of Prisoner Health* 2008;4:198–207.

34 Nijhawan AE, Salloway R, Nunn AS, Poshkus M, Clarke JG. Preventive healthcare for underserved women: results of a prison survey. *Journal of Women's Health* 2010;19:17–22.

35 Papadodima SA, Sakelliadis EI, Sergentanis TN, *et al.* Smoking in prison: a hierarchical approach at the crossroad of personality and childhood events. *European Journal of Public Health* 2010;20:470–4.

36 Plugge EH, Foster CE, Yudkin PL, Douglas N. Cardiovascular disease risk factors and women prisoners in the UK: the impact of imprisonment. *Health Promotion International* 2009;24:334–43.

37 Scottish Prison Service. *Prisoner Survey 2009*. Edinburgh: Scottish Prison Service, 2010.

38 Scottish Prison Service. *Female Offenders 2009*. Edinburgh: Scottish Prison Service, 2010.

39 Sieminska A, Jassem E, Konopa K. Prisoners' attitudes towards cigarette smoking and smoking cessation: a questionnaire study in Poland. *BMC Public Health* 2006;6:181.

40 Brooker C, Fox C, Barrett P, Syson-Nibbs L. A *Health Needs Assessment of Offenders on Probation Caseloads in Nottinghamshire & Derbyshire: Report of a Pilot Study*. Lincoln: CCAWI University of Lincoln, 2008.

41 Payne-James JJ, Green PG, Green N, Munro MHWM, Moore TCB. Healthcare issues of detainees in police custody in London, UK. *Journal of Forensic and Legal Medicine* 2010;17:11–17.

42 Singleton N, Meltzer H, Gatward R. *Psychiatric Morbidity among Prisoners*. London: Office of National Statistics, 1998.

43 Social Exclusion Unit. *Reducing Reoffending by Ex-prisoners*. London: Social Exclusion Unit, 2002.

44 Home Office. *National Reducing Re-offending Action Plan*. London: Home Office Communications Directorate, 2004.

45 Dooris M, Hunter D. *Organisations and Settings for Promoting Public Health*. London: Sage/Milton Keynes: Open University, 2007.

46 Prison Reform Trust. *Bromley Briefings Prison Factfile*. London: Prison Reform Trust, 2011.

47 Condon L, Hek G, Harris F. Choosing health in prison:Prisoners'views on making healthy choices in English prisons. *Health Education Journal* 2008;67:155–66.

48 Douglas N, Plugge E. A *Health Needs assessment for Women in Young Offender Institutions*. London: Youth Justice Board for England and Wales, 2006.

49 MacAskill S, Hayton P. *Stop Smoking Support in HM Prisons: The Impact of Nicotine Replacement Therapy*. Includes Best Practice Checklist. London: Department of Health; 2007.

50 Richmond RL, Butler T, Belcher JM, *et al.* Promoting smoking cessation among prisoners: feasibility of a multi-component intervention. *Australian and New Zealand Journal of Public Health* 2006;30:474–8.

51 Cropsey KL, Linker JA, Waite DE. An analysis of racial and sex differences for smoking among adolescents in a juvenile correctional centre. *Drug and Alcohol Dependence* 2008;92:156–63.

52 Wilcox SC. *Secondhand Smoke Signals from Prisons*. 105 edn. Michigan Law review, 2007.

53 Department of Corrections. Corrections News July/August 2012. Department of Corrections, 2012. www.corrections.govt.nz/__data/assets/pdf_file/0007/622888/ Correction_News_July_Aug_2012.pdf [Accessed 26 February 2013]

54 HM Prison Service. *Prison service Instruction 09/2007*. London: HM Prison Service, 2007.

55 Prison Office Association. *Health and Safety Smoke Free*. Prison Circular 157-2011. 2011.
56 Proescholdbell SK, Foley KL, Johnson J, Malek SH. Indoor air quality in prisons before and after implementation of a smoking ban law. *Tobacco Control* 2008;17:123–7.
57 Stuart GL, Meehan J, Moore TM, *et al*. Readiness to quit cigarette smoking, violence and psychopathology among arrested domestically violent men. *American Journal on Addictions* 2006;15:256–7.
58 Stuart GL, Meehan J, Temple JR, *et al*. Readiness to quit cigarette smoking, intimate partner violence, and substance abuse among arrested violent women. *American Journal on Addictions* 2006;15:396–9.
59 NHS Information Centre. *Statistics on Smoking: England, 2011*. London: The Health and Social Care Information Centre, 2011.
60 Eadie D, MacAskill S, McKell J, Baybutt M. Barriers and facilitators to a criminal justice tobacco control coordinator: an innovative approach to supporting smoking cessation among offenders. *Addiction* 2012;107:26–38.
61 Knox B, Black C, Hislop E. *Smoking Cessation in HMP Bowhouse, Kilmarnock*: Final Project Report. Ayr: Fresh Air-shire, NHS Ayrshire & Arran, 2006.
62 Jones L, Hayes F, MacAskill S, *et al*. *Evaluation of the impact of the PATH Support Fund – Final Report*. Edinburgh: PATH (Partnership Action on Tobacco and Health), 2007.
63 Platt S, Amos A, Bitel M, *et al*. *External Evaluation of the NHS Health Scotland/ASH Scotland Young People and Smoking Cessation Pilot Programme*. Edinburgh: NHS Health Scotland Online, 2009.
64 Cancer institute NSW. *Literature Review: Smoking and mental Ilness, other drug and alcohol addictions and prisons*. Sydney: Cancer Institute NSW, 2008.
65 Lincoln T, Tuthill RW, Roberts CA, *et al*. Resumption of smoking after release from a tobacco-free correctional facility. *Journal of Correctional Healthcare* 2009;15:190–16.
66 MacAskill S, Lindridge A, Stead M, *et al*. Social marketing with challenging target groups: Smoking cessation in prisons in England and Wales. *International Journal of Nonprofit and Voluntary Sector Marketing* 2008;13:251–61.
67 Lawrence S, Welfare H. The effects of the introduction of the non-smoking policy at HMYOI Warren Hill on bullying behaviour. *International Journal of Prisoner Health* 2008;4:134–45.
68 NHS Information Centre. *Statistics on alcohol: England, 2012*. London: NHS Information Centre, 2012.
69 McManus S, Meltzer H, Campion J. *Cigarette smoking and mental health in England. Data from the Adult Psychiatric Morbidity Survey*. London: National Centre for Social Research, 2010.
70 NHS Information Centre. *Statistics on drug misuse: England, 2012*. London: NHS Information Centre, 2012.
71 National Treatment Agency for Substance Misuse. *National and regional estimates of the prevalence of opiate and/or crack cocaine use 2008–09*. www.nta.nhs.uk/facts-prevalence.aspx [Accessed 26 February 2013]
72 Kalman D, Kim S, DiGirolamo G, Smelson D, Ziedonis D. Addressing tobacco use disorder in smokers in early remission from alcohol dependence: The case for integrating smoking cessation services in substance use disorder treatment programs. *Clinical Psychology Review* 2010;30:12–24.
73 Nahvi S, Richter K, Li X. Cigarette smoking and interest in quitting in methadone maintenance patients. *Addictive Behaviors* 2006;31:2127–34.
74 Green H, McGinnity A, Meltzer H, Ford T, Goodman R. *Mental Health of Children and Young People in Great Britain 2004*. London: Office of National Statistics, 2005.

75 Saraceno L, Munafò MR, Heron J. Genetic and non-genetic influences on the development of co-occurring alcohol problem use and internalizing symptomatology in adolescence: a review. *Addiction* 2009;104:1100–21.

76 Strandheim A, Holmen TL, Coombes L, Bentzen N. Alcohol intoxication and mental health among adolescents. A population review of 8983 young people, 13–19 years in North-Trøndelag, Norway: the Young-HUNT study. *Child and Adolescent Psychiatry and Mental Health* 2009;3:18.

77 Barnett J, Werners U, Secher SM. Substance use in a population-based clinic sample of people with first-episode psychosis. *British Journal of Psychiatry* 2007;190:515–20.

78 Compton WM, Thomas YF, Stinson FS, Grant BF. Prevalence, correlates, disability, and comorbidity of DSM-IV drug abuse and dependence in the United States: results from the National Epidemiologic Survey on Alcohol and Related Conditions. *Archives of General Psychiatry* 2007;64:566–76.

79 Drake R. Dual diagnosis. *Psychiatry* 2007;6:381–4.

80 Carra G, Johnson S. Variation in rates of comorbid substance misuse in psychosis between mental health settings and geographical areas in the UK. *Social Psychiatry and Psychiatric Epidemiology* 2009;44:429–47.

81 Hurt RD, Offord KP, Croghan IT, et al. Mortality following inpatient addictions treatment. Role of tobacco use in a community-based cohort. *Journal of the American Medical Association* 1996;275:1097–103.

82 Patkar AA, Sterling RC, Leone FT. Relationship between tobacco smoking and medical symptoms among cocaine-, alcohol-, and opiate-dependent patients. *American Journal on Addictions* 2002;11:209–18.

83 Gfroerer JC, Wu LT, Penne MA. *Initiation of Marijuana Use: Trends, Patterns, and Implications.* Analytic Series: A, 17th edn. Rockville, MD: Substance Abuse and Mental Health Services Administration, Office of Applied Studies, 2002.

84 US Department of Health and Human Services. *Preventing Tobacco Use Among Youth and Young Adults: A Report of the Surgeon General.* Washington DC: US Department of Health and Human Services 2012.

85 Ellickson PL, Hays RD, Bell RM. Stepping through the drug use sequence: longitudinal scalogram analysis of initiation and regular use. *Journal of Abnormal Psychology* 1992;101:441–51.

86 Yamaguchi K, Kandel DB. Patterns of drug use from adolescence to young adulthood: II. Sequences of progression. *American Journal of Public Health* 1984;74:668–72.

87 Tacke U, Wolff K, Finch E, Strang J. The effect of tobacco smoking on subjective symptoms of inadequacy ('not holding') of methadone dose among opiate addicts in methadone maintenance treatment. *Addiction Biology* 2001;6:137–45.

88 Frosch DL, Shoptaw S, Nahom D, Jarvik ME. Associations between tobacco smoking and illicit drug use among methadone-maintained opiate-dependent individuals. *Experimental and Clinical Psychopharmacology* 2000;8:97–103.

89 Frosch DL, Nahom D, Shoptaw S. Optimizing smoking cessation outcomes among the methadone maintained. *Journal of Substance Abuse Treatment* 2002;23:425–30.

90 Baca CT, Yahne CE. Smoking cessation during substance abuse treatment: What you need to know. *Journal of Substance Abuse Treatment* 2009;36:205–19.

91 Reichler H, Baker A, Lewin T. Smoking among in-patients with drug-related problems in an Australian psychiatric hospital. *Drug and Alcohol Review* 2001;20:231–7b.

92 Richter KP, Gibson CA, Ahluwalia JS. Tobacco use and quit attempts among methadone maintenance clients. *American Journal of Public Health* 2001;91:296–9.

93 Fuller BE, Guydish J, Tsoh J. Attitudes towards the integration of smoking cessation treatment into drug abuse clinics. *Journal of Substance Abuse Treatment,* 2007;32:53–60.

94 Harris J, Best D, Man L-H. Changes in cigarette smoking among alcohol and drug misusers during inpatient detoxification. *Addiction Biology* 2000;5:443–50.

95 Stimmel B, old M. Smoking and illicit drug use – a lesson yet to be learnt. *Journal of Addictive Diseases* 1998;17:1–5.

96 Prochaska JJ, Delucchi K, Hall SM. A meta-analysis of smoking cessation interventions with individuals in substance abuse treatment or recovery. *Journal of Consulting and Clinical Psychology* 2004;72:1144–1156.

97 Khara M, Okoli CTC. Smoking cessation outcomes among individuals with substance use and/or psychiatric disorder. *Journal of Addiction Research and Therapy* 2011;2:115.

98 Burling TA, Burling AS, Latini D. A controlled smoking cessation trial for substance-dependent inpatients. *Journal of Consulting and Clinical Psychology* 2001;69:295–304.

99 Department of Health. *Healthcare for Single Homeless People*. London: Office of the Chief Analyst, DH, 2010.

100 Reeve K, Batty E. The hidden truth about homelessness: Experiences of single homelessness in England. Crisis, 2012. www.crisis.org.uk/data/files/publications/HiddenTruthAboutHomelessness_web.pdf [Accessed 26 February 2013]

101 Crisis. Hidden *Homelessness. Britain's invisible city*. London: Crisis, 2004.

102 Bebbington PE, Bhugra D, Brugha T. Psychosis, victimisation and childhood disadvantage: evidence from the second British National Survey of Psychiatric Morbidity. *British Journal of Psychiatry* 2004;185:220–6.

103 Rees S. *Mental ill health in the adult single homeless population: a review of the literature*. London: Crisis, 2009.

104 St Mungo's. *Homelessness: it makes you sick. St Mungo's: opening doors for London's homeless*. London: ST Mungo's, 2008.

105 Craig T, Hodson S. Homeless youth in London: Childhood antecedents and psychiatric disorder. *Psychological Medicine* 1998;28:1388.

106 Maguire NJ, Johnson R, Vostanis P, Keats H, Remington RE. *Homelessness and complex trauma: a review of the literature*. Southampton: University of Southampton, 2009.

107 Homeless Link. The health and wellbeing of people who are homeless. Evidence from a national audit- interim report. 2010. www.ohrn.nhs.uk/resource/policy/HomelessHealthAudit.pdf [Accessed 26 February 2013]

108 Wincup E, Buckland G, Bayliss R. *Youth homelessness and substance misuse: report to the drugs and alcohol research unit*. London: Home Office Research, Development and Statistics Directorate, 2003.

109 Butler J, Okuyemi KS, Jean S. Smoking characteristics of a homeless population. *Substance Abuse* 2002;23:223–31.

110 Baggett TP, Rigotti NA. Cigarette smoking and advice to quit in a national sample of homeless adults. *American Journal of Preventive Medicine* 2010;39:164–72.

111 Thompson SJ. Risk/protective factors associated with substance use among runaway/homeless youth utilizing emergency shelter services nationwide. *Substance Abuse* 2004;25:13–26.

112 Connor SE, Cook RL, Herbert MI. Smoking cessation in a homeless population: There is a will, but is there a way? *Journal of General Internal Medicine* 2002;17:369–72.

113 Apollonio DE, Malone RE. Tobacco industry targeting of the homeless and mentally ill. *Tobacco Control* 2005;14:409–15.

114 Hwang SW, Wilkins R, Tjepkema M. Mortality among residents of shelters, rooming houses, and hotels in Canada: 11 year follow-up study. *British Medical Journal* 2009;339:b4036.

115 Health Development Agency. *Homelessness, Smoking and Health*. London: Health Development Agency, 2004.

116 Shelley D, Cantrell J, Wong S. Smoking cessation among sheltered homeless: A pilot. *American Journal of Health Behavior* 2010;34:544–52.

117 Okuyemi KS, Caldwell AR, Thomas JL. Homelessness and smoking cessation: Insights from focus groups. *Nicotine & Tobacco Research* 2006;8:287–96.

118 HM Government. *No health without mental health:a cross-government mental health outcomes strategy for people of all ages*. London: HMSO, 2011.

119 NICE. *How to stop smoking in pregnancy and following childbirth*. NICE public health guidance 26: *Quitting smoking in pregnancy and following childbirth*. London: NICE, 2010.

120 Royal College of Physicians. *Passive smoking and children: A report by the tobacco advisory group of the Royal College of Physicians*. London: RCP, 2010.

121 Brion MJ, Victoria C, Matijasevich A, *et al*. Maternal smoking and child psychological problems: disentangling causal and noncausal effects. *Pediatrics* 2010;126:57–65.

122 Ino T. Maternal smoking during pregnancy and offspring obesity: meta-analysis. *Pediatrics International* 2010;52:94–9.

123 Kwok P, Correy JF, Newman NM, Curran JT. Smoking and alcohol consumption during pregnancy: an epidemiological study in Tasmania. *Medical Journal of Australia* 1983;1:220–3.

124 Lumley J, Chamberlain C, Dodswell T, *et al*. Interventions for promoting smoking cessation during pregnancy. *Cochrane Database of Systematic Reviews* 2009;(3):CD001055.

125 LeClere FB, Wilson JB. Smoking Behaviour of recent mothers, 18–44 years of age, before and after pregnancy: United States, 1990. In: Va H (ed.), *Statistics*, 11th edn. Atlanta, GA: National Centre for Health Statistics, Centre for Disease Control, 1997.

126 Ershoff DH, Quinn VP, Boyd NR, Gregory M, Wirtschafter D. The Kiaser Permanent Prenatal Smoking-Cessation Trial- When more isn't better, what is enough? *American Journal of Preventive Medicine* 1999;17:161–8.

127 NHS Information Center for Health and Social Care. *Statistics on Women's Smoking Status at Time of Delivery: England, Quarter 3*. London: Health and Social Care Information Centre, Lifestyles Statistics, 2012.

128 Dejin-Karlsson E, Hanson BS, OPstergren PO, R*et al*. Psychosocial resources and persistent smoking in early pregnancy-a population study of women in their first pregnancy in Sweden. *Journal of Epidemiology and Community Health* 1996;50:33–9.

129 Flach C, Leese M, Heron J, *et al*. Antenatal domestic violence, maternal mental health and subsequent child behaviour: a cohort study. *British Journal of Obstetrics and Gynaecology* 2011;118:1383–91.

130 Goodwin R, Keyes K, Simuro N. Mental disorders and nicotine dependence among pregnant women in the United States. *Obstetrics and Gynecology* 2007;109:875–83.

131 Bick D, Howard L. When should women be screened for postnatal depression. *Expert Review in Neurotherapeutics* 2010;10:151–4.

132 Vesga-Lopez O, Blanco C, Keyes K, *et al*. Psychiatric Disorders in Pregnant and Postpartum Women in the United States. *Archives of General Psychiatry* 2008;65:10.

133 NICE. *Antenatal and Postnatal Mental Health: Clinical management and service guidance*. London: NICE, 2007.

134 Bennett HA, Einarson A, Taddio A, Oren G, Inarson TR. Prevalence of depression during pregnancy: Systematic review. *Obstetrics and Gynecology* 2004;103:698–709.

135 Grote NK, Bridge JA, Gavin AR, *et al*. A meta-analysis of depression during pregnancy and the risk of preterm birth, low birth weight, and intrauterine growth restriction. *Archives of General Psychiatry* 2010;67:1012–24.

136 Gold KJ, Dalton VK, Schwenk TL, Hayward RA. What causes pregnancy loss? Preexisting mental illness as an independent risk factor. *General Hospital Psychiatry* 2007;29:207–13.

137 Webb R, Abel K, Pickles A, Appleby L. Mortality in offspring of parents with psychotic disorders: a critical review and meta-analysis. *American Journal of Psychiatry* 2005;162:1045.

138 Howard LM, Kirkwood G, Latinovic R. Sudden infant death syndrome and maternal depression. *Journal of Clinical Psychiatry* 2007;68:1279–83.

139 Webb R, Wicks S, Dalman C, *et al*. Influence of environmental factors in higher risk of sudden infant death syndrome linked with parental mental illness. *Archives of General Psychiatry* 2010;67:69–77.

140 Shah N, Howard L. Screening for smoking and substance misuse in pregnant women with mental illness. *Psychiatric Bulletin* 2006;30:294–97.

141 Lewis SJ, Araya R, Davey Smith G, *et al*. Smoking is associated with, but does not cause, depressed mood in pregnancy – a mendelian randomization study. *PloS ONE* 2011;6.

142 Munafo MR, Heron J, Araya R. Smoking patterns during pregnancy and postnatal period and depressive symptoms. *Nicotine and Tobacco Research* 2008;10:1609–20.

143 Coleman T, Cooper S, Thornton JG, *et al*. Smoking, Nicotine, and Pregnancy (SNAP) Trial Team. A randomized trial of nicotine-replacement therapy patches in pregnancy. *New England Journal of Medicine* 2012;366:808–18.

144 Taylor T, Hajek P. *Smoking Cessation Services for Pregnant Women*. London: Health Development Agency, 2001.

145 American Congress of Obstetricians and Gynecologists. Smoking cessation during pregnancy. Committee Opinion Number 471, 2010. www.acog.org/Resources_And_Publications/Committee_Opinions/Committee_on_Health_Care_for_Underserved_Women/Smoking_Cessation_During_Pregnancy [Accessed 26 February 2013]

146 Howard LM, Bekele D, Rowe M, *et al*. Smoking cessation in pregnant women with mental disorders: a cohort and nested qualitative study. *British Journal of Obstetrics and Gynaecology* 2013;120:362–70.

147 Howard LM, Goss C, Leese M, Thornicroft G. Medical outcome of pregnancy in women with psycotic disorders and their infants in the first year after birth. *British Journal of Psychiatry* 2003;182:63–7.

148 Aubin HJ, Rollema H, Svensson TH, Winterer G. Smoking, quitting, and psychiatric disease: a review. *Neuroscience and Biobehavioural Reviews* 2012;36:271–84.

149 Brown R, Kahler C, Niaura R. Cognitive-behavioral treatment for depression in smoking cessation. *Journal of Consulting Clinical Psychology* 2001;69:471–80.

150 Haas AL, Munoz RF, Humfleet GL, Reus VI, Hall SM. Influences of mood, depression history and treatment modality on outcomes in smoking cessation. *Journal of Consulting Clinical Psychology* 2004;72:563–70.

151 Pickett K, Wakschlag L, Dai L, Leventhal B. Fluctuations of maternal smoking during pregnancy. *Obstetrics and Gynecology* 2003;101:140–7.

152 McNally L, Oyefeso A, Annan J, *et al*. A survey of staff attitudes to smoking-related policy and intervention in psychiatric and general health care settings. *Journal of Public Health* 2006;28:192–6.

153 El-Mohandes AA, El-Khorazaty MN, Kiely M, Gantz MG. Smoking cessation and relapse among pregnant African-American smokers in Washington, DC. *Maternal and Child Health Journal* 2011;15:S96–105.

154 El-Mohandes AA, Kiely M, Blake SM, Gantz MG, El-Khorazaty MN. An intervention to reduce environmental tobacco smoke exposure improves pregnancy outcomes. *Pediatrics* 2010;125:721–8.

155 Cincirpini PM, Blalock JA, Minnix JA, et al. Effects of an intensive depression-focused intervention for smoking cessation in pregnancy. *Journal of Consulting Clinical Psychology* 2010;78:44–54.

156 Lewis G. Saving mothers' lives: reviewing maternal deaths to make motherhood safer: 2006–08. *BJOG: An International Journal of Obstetrics & Gynaecology* 2011;118:1–203.

157 Cornelius MD, Day NL. Developmental consequences of prenatal tobacco exposure. *Current Opinion in Neurology* 2009;22:121–5.

158 Ekblad M, Gissler M, Lehtonen L, Korkeila J. Prenatal smoking exposure and the risk of psychiatric morbidity into young adulthood. *Archives of General Psychiatry* 2010;67:841–9.

159 Ashford J, Lier PACV. Prenatal smoking and internalizing and externalizing problems in children studied from childhood to late adolescence. *American Academy of Child and Adolescent Psychiatry* 2008;47:779–87.

160 Bandiera FC, Richardson AK, Lee DJ, et al. Secondhand smoke exposure and mental health among children and adolescents. *Archives of Pediatric and Adolescent Medicine* 2011;165:332–8.

161 Hamer M, Ford T, Stamatakis E, Dockray S, Batty DG. Objectively measured secondhand smoke exposure and mental health in children: Evidence from the Scottish Health Survey. *Archives of Pediatric and Adolescent Medicine* 2011;165:326–31.

162 Twardella D, Bolte G, Fromme H, Wildner MvKR. Exposure to secondhand tobacco smoke and child behaviour – results from a cross-sectional study among preschool children in Bavaria. *Acta Paediatrica* 2010;99:106–11.

163 Cho S-C, Kim B-N, Hong Y-C, et al. Effect of environmental exposure to lead and tobacco smoke on inattentive and hyperactive symptoms and neurocognitive performance in children. *Journal of Children* 2010;51:1050–7.

164 Salvo EPD, Liu YH, Brenner S, Weitzman M. Adult household smoking is associated with increased child emotional and behavioural problems. *Journal of Developmental and Behavioral Pediatrics* 2010;31:107–15.

165 Lawrence D, Mitrou F, Sawyer MG, et al. Smoking status, mental disorders and emotional and behavioural problems in young people: child and adolescent component of the National Survey of Mental Health and Wellbeing. *Australian and New Zealand Journal of Psychiatry* 2010;44:805–14.

166 Chaiton M, Cohen J, O'Loughlin J, Rehm J, et al. A systematic review of longitudinal studies on the association between depression and smoking in adolescents. *BMC Public Health* 2009;9:356.

167 Millberger S, Biederman J, Faraone SV, Chen L, Jones J. ADHD isassociated with early initiation of cigarette smoking in children and adolescents. *Journal of the American Academy of Child and Adolescent Psychiatry* 1997;36:37–44.

168 Glass K, Flory K. Why does ADHD confer risk for cigarette smoking? A review of psychosocial mechanisms. *Clinical Child and Family Psychology Review* 2010;13:291–313.

169 Lambert N. The contribution of childhood ADHD, conduct problems, and stimulant treatment to adolescent and adult tobacco and psychoactive substance use. *Ethical Human Psychology and Psychiatry* 2005;7:197–221.

170 Whalen CK, Henker B, Gehricke J-G, King PS. Is there a link between adolescent cigarette smoking and pharmacotherapy for ADHD? *Psychology of Addictive Behaviours* 2003;17:332–5.

171 Modesto-Lowe V, Danforth J, Neering C, Easton C. Can we prevent smoking in children with ADHD: a review of the literature. *Connecticut Medicine* 2010;74:229–36.

172 Cawley J, Markowitz S, Tauras J. Lighting up and slimming down: the effects of body weight and cigarette prices on adolescent smoking initiation. *Journal of Health Economics* 2004;23:293–311.

173 Potter BK, Pederson LL. Does a relationship exist between body weight, concerns about weight, and smoking among adolescents? An integration of the literature with an emphasis on gender. *Nicotine and Tobacco Research* 2004;6:397–425.

174 Wiseman CV, Turco RM, Sunday SR, Halmi KA. Smoking and body image concerns in adolescent girls. *International Journal of Eating Disorders* 1998;24:429–33.

175 Ford T, Vostanis P, Meltzer H, Goodman R. Psychiatric disorder amongst British children looked after by local authorities; comparision with children living in private households. *British Journal of Psychiatry* 2007;190:319–25.

176 Meltzer H, Corbin T, Goodman R, Ford T. *The Mental Health of Young people Looked After by Local Authorities in England*. London: Office of National Statistics, 2003.

177 Meltzer H, Goodman R, Ford T. *Mental Health of Children and Adolescents in Great Britain*. London: Office of National Statistics, 2000.

178 Ridley J, McCluskey S. Exploring the perceptions of young people in care and care leavers of their health needs. *Scottish Journal of Residential Child Care* 2003;55–65.

179 Friel B, Parsons L. Smoking cessation and looked after and accommodated children. National Smoking Cessation Conference 14–15th June 2010.

180 MacMillan I. *Smoke Free Care Placements for Looked After and Accommodated Children and Young People*. Glasgow City Council/NHS Greater Glasgow and Clyde, 2007.

181 Jackson S, McParlin P. The education of children in care. *The Psychologist* 2006;19:90–3.

182 Scott J, Hill M. *The Health of Looked After and Accommodated Children in Scotland*. Edinburgh: Social Work Inspection Agency, 2006.

183 Ward H, Jones H, Lynch M, Skuse T. Issues concerning the health of looked after children. *Adoption and Fostering* 2002;26:8–18.

184 Department for Education and Skills. *Care Matters: Time for change*. London: Department for Education and Skills, 2007.

185 Royal College of Psychiatrists. *Physical health in mental health: report of a scoping group*. OP67. London: RCP, 2009.

186 National Insitute for Health and Clinical Excellence. *Smoking cessation services in primary care, pharmacies, local authorities and workplace, particularly for manual working groups, pregnant women and hard to reach communities*. PH 10. London: NICE, 008.

187 Price JH, Sidani JE, Price JA. Child and adolescent psychiatrists' practices in assisting their adolescent patients who smoke to quit smoking. *Journal of the American Academy of Child and Adolescent Psychiatry* 2007;46:60–7.

188 National Children's Bureau. *Healthy Care E-briefing*, April 2007. www.ncb.org.uk/media/177337/supporting_and_training_foster_carers_to_promote_health_and_well-being.pdf [Accessed 26 February 2013]

8 | The economic cost of smoking in people with mental disorders

8.1 Introduction

In the UK in 2009–10 the cost imposed on society as a result of the health- and social care costs, human costs and output losses attributable to mental disorders were estimated at over £105bn.[1,2] In the same year, mental health services accounted for approximately 14% of the annual NHS budget.[3] The economic burden of smoking is estimated at over £14bn in total costs to society, including over £5bn to the NHS, each year.[4] Mental disorders and smoking therefore both impose substantial economic burdens on healthcare services and wider society, but, in contrast to those of mental disorders alone, the costs of smoking are entirely preventable. This chapter aims to estimate the economic costs to the NHS of smoking among people with mental disorders. Annual costs associated with smoking in patients with mental disorders in the UK were assessed from the NHS personal social services (PSS) perspective, based on the population estimates of the number of people in the UK with mental disorders and the numbers of those who smoke, presented in Chapter 2. All costs are estimated in pounds sterling for the 2009–10 financial year.

8.2 Estimating the costs of diseases caused by smoking in people with mental disorders

Smoking causes or exacerbates many diseases, but most of the mortality and morbidity caused by smoking at population level arise from effects on the risk of lung cancer, cardiovascular disease and chronic obstructive pulmonary disease.[5,6] To estimate the ensuing economic costs of healthcare provision for diseases caused by smoking in people with mental disorders, we have used the attributable risk approach[7,8] as originally devised by Levin,[9] and tailored and widely used in the estimation of smoking-attributable health outcomes.[5,10–12] The proportion of disease attributable to smoking in current and former smokers compared with never smokers is estimated from the relative risks of disease and prevalence of exposure using the following formula:

$$\mathrm{AP} = \frac{p_{\mathrm{cur}}\,(r_{\mathrm{cur}} - 1) + p_{\mathrm{ex}}\,(r_{\mathrm{ex}} - 1)}{1 + p_{\mathrm{cur}}\,(r_{\mathrm{cur}} - 1) + p_{\mathrm{ex}}\,(r_{\mathrm{ex}} - 1)}$$

where AP is the attributable proportion, p_{cur} is the proportion who are current smokers, r_{cur} the relative risk for current compared with never smokers, p_{ex} the proportion who are ex-smokers and r_{ex} the relative risk for ex- compared with never smokers.

The attributable proportion is then multiplied by aggregated numbers of hospital admissions by diseases, outpatient visits, consultations and prescriptions for relevant diseases to generate an estimate of the amount of resource use attributable to smoking. Finally, smoking-attributable costs are calculated by multiplying the attributable use of healthcare services by estimated unit costs.

To provide conservative estimates we have assumed that smoking increases mortality by increasing the incidence of disease rather than worsening case fatality among patients who would already be affected by the disease. Although higher risks of cardiovascular disease have been reported in people with severe mental illness[13] we have also assumed for the purposes of economic evaluation that mental disorders do not of themselves appreciably increase the incidence or severity of smoking-related diseases across the wider population of people with mental disorders.

8.3 Hospital costs of treating disease caused by smoking in people with mental disorders

Tables 8.1 and 8.2 list fatal and non-fatal diseases caused by smoking, their ICD-10 (*International classification of disease*, 10th revision) codes, and the relative risks for developing each disease for current and former smokers compared with never smokers, by gender. Spontaneous abortion is included with non-fatal diseases. The relative risks for fatal diseases were taken from *Statistics on smoking: England, 2010* which followed the estimation of smoking-attributable mortality in the Health Profile of England (HPE) published in 2007.[8,10] Relative risks for non-fatal diseases and spontaneous abortion were as originally used in Wald and Hackshaw's epidemiological overview[14] and updated in later reports.[5,10,15]

Hospital admission data for each disease were obtained from the Hospital Episode Statistics (HES) for England during the period April 2009 to March 2010,[17] as the total number of hospital admissions (finished consultant episodes or FCEs) for each diagnosis, and from equivalent sources for Wales, Scotland and Northern Ireland.[18–20] Costs for hospital admissions were estimated as a weighted average of ordinary admissions (elective, non-elective) and day cases, taken from the relevant healthcare resource groups (HRGs) in the 2009–10 NHS

Table 8.1 Relative risks for fatal diseases in current and ex-smokers compared with never smokers, by gender

Disease caused by smoking	ICD-10 code	Age	Male smokers Current (r_{cur})	Ex (r_{ex})	Female smokers Current (r_{cur})	Ex (r_{ex})
Malignant neoplasms						
Lip, oral cavity, pharynx	C00–C14	35+	10.89	3.40	5.08	2.29
Oesophagus	C15	35+	6.76	4.46	7.75	2.79
Stomach	C16	35+	1.96	1.47	1.36	1.32
Pancreas	C25	35+	2.31	1.15	2.25	1.55
Larynx	C32	35+	14.60	6.34	13.02	5.16
Trachea, lung, bronchus	C33–C34	35+	23.26	8.70	12.69	4.53
Cervix uteri	C53	35+	1.00	1.00	1.59	1.14
Kidney and renal pelvis	C64–C66, C68	35+	2.50	1.70	1.40	1.10
Urinary bladder	C67	35+	3.27	2.09	2.22	1.89
Malignant neoplasm without specification of site	C80	35+	4.40	2.50	2.20	1.30
Myeloid leukaemia	C92	35+	1.80	1.40	1.20	1.30
Cardiovascular diseases						
Ischaemic heart disease	I20–I25	35–54	4.20	2.00	5.30	2.60
		55–64	2.50	1.60	2.80	1.10
		65–74	1.80	1.30	2.10	1.20
		75+	1.40	1.10	1.40	1.20
Other heart disease	I00–I09, I26–I51		1.78	1.22	1.49	1.14
Cerebrovascular disease	I60–I69	35–54	4.40	1.10	5.40	1.30
		55–64	3.10	1.10	3.70	1.30
		65–74	2.20	1.10	2.60	1.30
		75+	1.60	1.10	1.30	1.00
Atherosclerosis	I70	35+	2.44	1.33	1.83	1.00
Aortic aneurysm	I71	35+	6.21	3.07	7.07	2.07
Other arterial diseases	I72–I78	35+	2.07	1.01	2.17	1.12
Respiratory diseases						
Pneumonia, influenza	J10–J18	35–64	2.50	1.40	4.30	1.10
		65+	2.00	1.40	2.20	1.10
Bronchitis, emphysema	J40–J42, J43	35+	17.10	15.64	12.04	11.77
Chronic airway obstruction	J44	35+	10.58	6.80	13.08	6.78
Digestive diseases						
Stomach ulcer, duodenal ulcer	K25–K27	35+	5.40	1.80	5.50	1.40

Source: *Profile of England, 2007* and *Statistics on smoking: England, 2010*.[10,16]

Table 8.2 Relative risks for non-fatal diseases and spontaneous abortion for current and ex-smokers

Disease caused by smoking	ICD-10 code	Current smokers (r_{cur})	Ex-smokers (r_{ex})
Crohn's disease	K50	2.10	1.00
Periodonitis	K05	3.97	1.68
Age-related cataract (45+)	H25	1.54	1.11
Hip fracture 55–64	S72.0–S72.21	1.17	1.02
Hip fracture 65–74	S72.0–S72.21	1.41	1.08
Hip fracture 75+ male	S72.0–S72.21	1.76	1.14
Hip fracture 75+ female	S72.0–S72.21	1.85	1.22
Spontaneous abortion (smoking during pregnancy)	O03	1.28	1

Source: Statistics on smoking: England, 2010.[10]

reference costs,[21,22] by linking disease ICD codes to the most recent HRG4 groups.[23] From these data we estimate that, in the financial year 2009–10, there were 2.6 million FCEs among adults aged over 35 with mental health problems in the UK that were attributable to smoking (Table 8.3).

Applying NHS reference costs to these smoking-attributable inpatient episodes yields an estimated hospital admission cost of £352m (£166m for males, £186m for females). Table 8.4 lists the estimated hospital costs by disease group and gender, and demonstrates (as expected) that malignancy, cardiovascular and respiratory diseases are the dominant sources of attributable costs. Figure 8.1 provides the breakdown of costs by mental disorder, and demonstrates that the great majority of costs arise from people with anxiety and/or depression.

Table 8.3 Number of hospital admissions by countries: UK 2009–10

	Finished consultant episodes (FCEs)	FCEs attributable to smoking among people with mental disorders	Source
England	16,806,196	2,346,078	HES online
Wales	892,655	124,611	PEDW
Scotland	639,111	89,217	ISD Scotland
Northern Ireland	583,501	81,454	HSC: Health and Social Care in Northern Ireland
Sum	18,921,463	2,641,361	

Smoking and mental health

Table 8.4 Estimated costs of hospital admissions attributable to smoking in people with mental disorders, UK 2009–10

Diseases that can be caused by smoking	Female	Male	All adults
Malignant neoplasms	£64,522,066	£46,134,951	£110,657,017
Cardiovascular diseases	£52,479,070	£56,217,925	£108,696,994
Respiratory diseases	£36,881,429	£58,070,523	£94,951,952
Digestive diseases	£4,935,875	£5,296,468	£10,232,343
Non-fatal diseases	£6,916,386	£20,737,207	£27,653,593
Total cost	£165,734,826	£186,457,073	£352,191,899

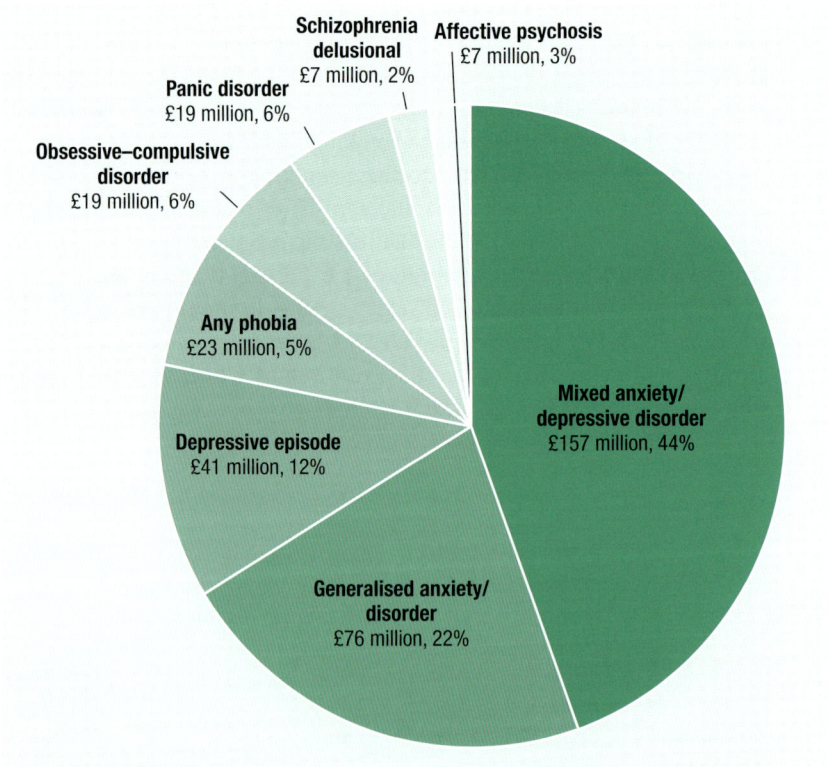

Fig 8.1 Breakdown of total inpatient costs due to smoking in mental health.

8.4 Outpatient services and primary care

Outpatient and primary care use attributable to smoking in people with mental disorders were estimated using generic NHS service use data, taking relative risk estimates of service use in current and ex-smokers relative to non-smokers from a recent study by Callum and colleagues, in turn based on data reported in the 2006 General Household Survey (GHS)[5] (Table 8.5).

Data on GP and practice nurse consultations were obtained from the QResearch database, which estimates that the total number of consultations in England in 2008 was 300.4 million, of which 62% and 34% respectively were undertaken by GPs and nurses.[24] During 2010 an estimated £9bn was spent by the NHS in England on prescription drugs in primary care, and 98% of these drugs were prescribed by GPs.[25] In 2010 a total of 927 million prescription items were dispensed, with an average net ingredient cost per prescription item of £9.53.[26] Average costs for GP and nurse visits were sourced from the Personal Social Services Research Unit (PSSRU) unit costs 2010, quantified at £32 per GP consultation and £10 per practice nurse consultation.[27] As there are no direct sources of data on the number of GP and practice nurse consultations and prescriptions outside England, we used the data for England to extrapolate costs for the UK, based on mid-2010 population estimates from the Office for National Statistics (ONS).[28] Data on outpatient attendances were obtained from HES data.[17] In 2009–10, the number of outpatient attendances for adults aged 35 and over was 27 million for males and 21 million for females. According to NHS reference cost data, the average cost of an adult outpatient visit in 2009–10 was £98.[22] Data for Wales, Scotland and Northern Ireland were obtained from the Health and Care statistics on the Welsh government website, ISD of National Services Scotland and NWIS websites respectively.[29–31]

Table 8.6 lists the number of outpatient and primary care attendances and prescriptions issued in primary care that are attributable to smoking among

Table 8.5 Relative risk (RR) estimates for outpatient and primary care service use based on reports of health service use, General Household Survey, 2006

	Current smokers		Ex-smokers	
	RR	95% CI	RR	95% CI
GP consultations	1.18	1.03–1.34	1.35	1.21–1.50
GP prescriptions	1.28	1.08–1.51	1.31	1.14–1.50
Practice nurse consultations	1.11	0.91–1.37	1.37	1.18–1.60
Outpatient attendances	1.05	0.88–1.24	1.17	1.01–1.37

CI, confidence interval.
Source: Callum et al., 2010.[5]

Table 8.6 Smoking-attributable costs for outpatient attendance and primary care among mental health patients

	Male		Female		All adults			
	No. of activities	Costs	No. of activities	Costs	No. of activities	Costs	No. of activities	Costs
GP consultations	1,250,664	£41,071,804	1,863,256	£61,189,323	3,113,920	£102,261,127		
GP prescriptions	7,419,253	£70,705,483	11,361,460	£108,274,711	18,780,713	£178,980,193		
Practice nurse consultations	572,186	£5,721,864	828,437	£8,284,366	1,400,623	£14,006,230		
Outpatient attendances	358,997	£35,181,734	367,940	£36,058,093	726,937	£71,239,828		
Total	9,601,101	£152,680,885	14,421,092	£213,806,493	24,022,193	£366,487,378		

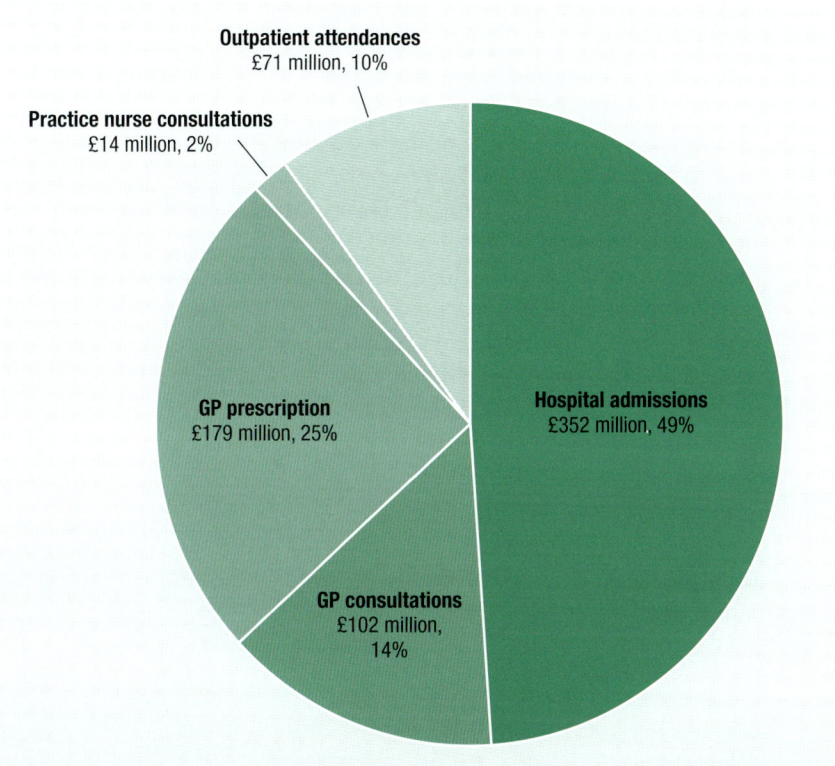

Fig 8.2 Breakdown of costs due to smoking-related diseases to the NHS among people with mental disorders [Figures may not sum to total due to rounding].

people with mental disorders in 2009–10, and their estimated costs. In total, 0.7 million outpatient visits were attributable to smoking among people with mental disorders, at a cost to the NHS of £71m. The number of GP consultations, nurse consultations and GP prescriptions attributable to smoking are 3 million, 1 million and 19 million respectively, and generate a total primary care cost of £295m per year. In contrast to hospital admission costs, these primary care and outpatient costs were higher for females than for males.

Figure 8.2 summarises the total overall estimated costs to the NHS of diseases caused by smoking in people with mental disorders. The total was £719m, of which just under half was the result of inpatient episodes.

8.5 Cost savings from psychotropic drug dose reduction after smoking cessation

As smoking increases the metabolism of some psychotropic drugs, smoking cessation can result in appreciable reductions in drug dose requirements (see

Chapter 5) and hence generate cost savings. Table 8.7 lists a selection of psychotropic drugs affected by smoking in this way, together with the best-case, maximum percentage dose reduction needed with smoking cessation, as taken from the Maudsley prescribing guidelines.[32]

For patients prescribed one or more psychoactive medications, drug prescriptions to smokers and non-smokers in 1 year were derived from the THIN (The Health Improvement Network) dataset (see Chapter 2), and unit costs for each drug by different dose forms and strength sourced from NHS prescription costs.[33] Cost savings from stopping smoking were then calculated by multiplying the percentage dose reduction by the dose used in smokers, and corresponding unit costs. In total, quitting smoking among people with mental health disorders has the potential to save the NHS £40m per year in psychotropic medicine costs. The greatest cost savings are from proprietary

Table 8.7 Drug cost saving from reduced doses by stopping smoking

Drug	Best-case percentage dose reduction with smoking cessation	Smoking prevalence (%)	Cost saving
Clozapine	50	51.5	£136,000
Duloxetine	50	32.5	£3,314,000
Fluphenazine	50	40.3	£106,000
Fluvoxamine	33	28.7	£43,000
Haloperidol	20	25.5	£865,000
Olanzapine	50	40.7	£26,710,000
Anxiolytic benzodiazepines			
Diazepam	50	29.4	£1,926,000
Alprazolam	50	22.8	£13,000
Chlordiazepoxide	50	52.4	£286,000
Oxazepam	50	27.7	£329,000
Lorazepam	50	22.7	£1,244,000
Tricyclic antidepressants			
Amitriptyline	50	22.5	£2,395,000
Clomipramine	50	26.9	£534,000
Dosulepin	50	24.3	£651,000
Doxepin	50	19.8	£58,000
Imipramine	50	20.8	£114,000
Lofepramine	50	28.2	£529,000
Nortriptyline	50	19.7	£391,000
Trimipramine	50	20.3	£239,000
Total cost saving			**£39,882,000**

olanzapine (£27m) and duloxetine (£3m), although the availability since 2011 of non-proprietary olanzapine at a cost of around 30% of the proprietary form[34] would reduce the potential savings, if all prescribed olanzapine were non-proprietary, to £9m.

8.6 Life-years gained from smoking cessation in mental disorders

Smoking cessation substantially increases life expectancy. Half of smokers die prematurely, unless they quit,[35] and quitting smoking at age 30, 40, 50 or 60 years gains, respectively, about 10, 9, 6 and 3 years of additional life expectancy.[36] Recent data from the NHS Health and Social Care Information Centre (HSCIC) indicate that mortality in people with serious mental disorder is three times the population average.[37]

Taking data from the Adult Psychiatric Morbidity Survey (APMS) in England,[38] in combination with mid-2009 UK population estimates published by the Office for National Statistics[39] and smoking prevalence by mental health diagnosis from Table 2.3 (see Chapter 2), we have estimated the numbers of smokers with these mental disorders, by age, in the UK (Table 8.8).

As the majority of people with mental disorders are diagnosed by their mid-20s,[40] their life-years gained (LYG) by stopping smoking can be assumed to be the same as for the general population. Table 8.8 shows estimated LYG by smoking cessation for individuals with mental disorders by age, with discounting to reflect individuals' and society's time preference[41,42] at 3.5% per annum, in line with the methods of technology appraisal recommended by the National Institute for Health and Clinical Excellence (NICE).[43]

Table 8.9 presents the estimated LYG for a range of smoking cessation rates among people with mental health diagnoses in the UK. Achieving cessation in 25%, 50% or 100% of people with mental disorders will result in a gain of 5.5 million, 11 million and 22 million undiscounted life-years, respectively. The corresponding discounted LYG figures, at a 3.5% discount rate, are 1.4, 2.7 and 5.4 million.

Smoking cessation is one of the most cost-effective lifesaving public health or medical interventions.[44–48] When only comparing the costs of an intervention with no intervention, the estimated incremental cost per quality-adjusted life-year (QALY) gained varies from around £221 to around £9,515.[49] Even if we assume that the effectiveness of smoking cessation interventions for people with mental health disorders is only half that observed in the general population, smoking cessation is still highly cost-effective when compared with the NICE willingness-to-pay threshold of £20,000–£30,000 per QALY.[43]

Table 8.8 Number of smokers with mental disorders by age in the UK[38]

Mental disorder	16–24	25–34	35–44	45–54	55–64	65–74	75+	All
Depressive episode	45,467	50,057	71,432	89,669	37,980	15,467	19,955	333,187
Phobias	32,883	47,404	55,715	37,393	31,140	5,700	1,764	214,702
Generalised anxiety disorder	69,610	89,482	22,686	35,972	79,333	46,171	33,644	579,943
Obsessive–compulsive disorder	48,031	34,362	27,320	27,807	11,424	4,630	5,797	157,490
Panic disorder	16,783	26,186	24,132	16,461	14,969	5,776	4,763	112,967
Mixed anxiety and depression	166,084	189,673	164,610	209,184	126,609	74,764	62,364	992,480
Probable psychosis	10,310	11,192	29,478	20,240	11,625	2,116	–	99,767
Post-traumatic stress disorder	98,695	84,014	81,241	93,705	39,448	17,083	7,769	423,800
Attention deficit hyperactivity disorder	21,654	14,625	21,738	15,253	4,019	–	1,611	82,836
Eating disorder	46,371	30,700	22,052	29,756	6,603	4,370	521	141,146
All	555,888	577,696	620,404	675,441	363,150	176,078	138,190	3,138,317[a]

[a]Discrepancy with Table 2.5 due to rounding errors.

Table 8.9 Life-years gained (LYG) by stopping smoking at different age groups

Age at quitting	Individual[a]	Discount rate (%)	Discounted until age	Individual discounted LYG	Population LYG from smoking cessation among people with mental health diagnoses at given quit rate percentage in people with mental disorders					
					Undiscounted LYG			Discounted LYG		
					25%	50%	100%	25%	50%	100%
<35	10	3.5	80	1.67	2,833,959	5,667,918	11,335,836	507,430	1,014,860	2,029,720
35–44	9	3.5	80	2.12	1,395,909	2,791,818	5,583,635	352,568	705,136	1,410,272
45–54	6	3.5	80	2.00	1,013,162	2,026,324	4,052,649	360,968	721,936	1,443,871
55–64	3	3.5	80	1.41	272,363	544,725	1,089,451	136,880	273,760	547,521
Total					5,515,393	11,030,786	22,061,572	1,357,846	2,715,693	5,431,385

[a]Data from Doll et al.[36]

8.7 Harm reduction approaches

Given the high rates of smoking and low rates of cessation in people with mental disorders to date, effective harm reduction strategies, such as providing safe medicinal nicotine products, have great potential as acceptable long-term or even lifelong substitutes for smoking.[50] We have estimated the order of magnitude of lifetime harm reduction in this population, using as examples the costs of two currently widely used nicotine replacement therapy (NRT) products, nicotine transdermal patches and nicotine inhalators. In so doing we have assumed an average cigarette consumption of 19 cigarettes/day among smokers with mental disorders,[51] and that to replace fully the 1 mg nicotine delivered to the circulation by each cigarette,[52] at 50% bioavailability,[53] 40 mg NRT will be required each day. The average net ingredient cost for 40 mg NRT is approximately £3.00 for nicotine patches and £1.40 for inhalators.[26]

As data comparing quality of life between long-term medicinal nicotine users and cigarette smokers are limited,[54] we have assumed that as tobacco smoke, rather than nicotine itself, is responsible for most of the adverse health effects of smoking, smokers who switch completely to using NRT products will get the same health benefits as those who quit all smoking and nicotine use.[55] Health benefits gained were measured using LYG and expected QALYs.[41] Both costs and health benefits were discounted at 3.5% per annum following NICE recommendations.[43] Table 8.10 presents the lifetime costs and health benefits of using nicotine patches and inhalators as substitutes for smoking, and the corresponding cost-effectiveness ratios for a number of different age ranges. Assuming that 2.5% of people who use NRT will quit all nicotine use entirely each year, the discounted lifetime cost was estimated as £16,711 per person for nicotine patches and £7,569 per person for inhalators (Table 8.10). If all current smokers with a mental disorder switched their smoking to NRT products immediately, over 1 million life-years will be gained for the group as a whole. The cost per LYG is £8,629 for nicotine patches and £3,908 for nicotine inhalators.

The Cochrane review of NRT in smoking cessation shows discounted QALY gains for a successful lifetime quitter, compared with one who continues smoking, to be 2.22, 2.58, 2.14 and 0.99 for people who stop smoking at age 30, 40, 50 and 60, respectively.[56] In total, 1.1 million QALYs will be gained if 100% of the smokers using NRT products were to replace tobacco smoking with alternative forms of nicotine delivery immediately. Based on the above assumptions, a cost-effectiveness ratio of £7,956 per QALY gained for nicotine patches and £3,603 per QALY for inhalators has been estimated. These results indicate that substituting nicotine from smoking cigarettes with either nicotine patches or nicotine inhalators is a cost-effective strategy compared with continuing smoking, given willingness-to-pay thresholds of £20,000–£30,000 per additional QALY gained.[43] The earlier an individual substitutes smoking for a harm reduction alternative, the more cost-effective the strategy becomes.

Table 8.10 Lifetime cost and health benefits using harm reduction strategies

Age group	<35	35–44	45–54	55–64	Total
Number of smokers with mental health disorders, UK	211,755	108,942	130,407	74,455	525,560
Discounted cost of lifetime nicotine patch/person	£18,083	£17,399	£15,870	£13,276	£16,711
Discounted cost of lifetime nicotine inhalator/person	£8,191	£7,881	£7,188	£6,013	£7,569
Discounted LYG per quitter	1.79	2.27	2.14	1.51	
Discounted QALY gain per quitter	2.22	2.58	2.14	0.99	
LYG (lifetime substitution in 25% of the mental health population)	2,833,959	1,395,909	1,013,162	272,363	5,515,393
LYG (lifetime substitution in 50% of the mental health population)	5,667,918	2,791,818	2,026,324	544,725	11,030,785
LYG (lifetime substitution in 100% of the mental health population)	11,335,836	5,583,635	4,052,649	1,089,451	22,061,571
Cost/LYG (patch)	£10,099	£7,654	£7,424	£8,806	£8,629

LYG, life-years gained; QUALY, quality-adjusted life-year.

8.8 Summary

> The NHS spends approximately £720m per annum in primary and secondary care treating smoking-related disease in people with mental disorders.
> These costs arise from an annual estimated 2.6 million avoidable hospital admissions, 3.1 million GP consultations and 18.8 million prescriptions.
> The majority of these service costs arise from people diagnosed with anxiety and/or depression.
> Smoking increases psychotropic drug costs in the UK by up to £40m per annum.
> Achieving cessation in 25%, 50% and 100% of people with mental disorders would respectively result in a gain of 5.5 million, 11 million and 22 million undiscounted life-years in the UK. At 3.5% discounting, the corresponding figures are 1.4, 2.7 and 5.4 million life-years gained.
> Harm reduction through lifelong substitution with medicinal nicotine is highly cost-effective when compared with continuing smoking, at around £8,000 per QALY gained for lifetime nicotine patch use and £3,600 per QALY for inhalators.
> Addressing the high prevalence of smoking in people with mental disorders offers the potential to realise substantial cost savings to the NHS, as well as benefits in quantity and quality of life.

References

1 Cyhlarova E, McCulloch A, McGuffin P, Wykes T. *Economic burden of mental illness cannot be tackled without research investment*. London: Mental Health Foundation, 2010.
2 Centre for Mental Health. *The economic and social costs of mental health problems in 2009/10*. London: Centre for Mental Health, 2010.
3 Department of Health. Departmental Report 2009: *The Health and Personal Social Services Programmes*. www.official-documents.gov.uk/document/cm75/7593/7593.pdf [Accessed 12 November 2012]
4 Allender S, Balakrishnan R, Scarborough P, al. The burden of smoking-related ill health in the UK. *Tobacco Control* 2009;18:262–7.
5 Callum C, White P. *Tobacco in London: The preventable burden*. London: SmokeFree London and The London Health Observatory, 2004.
6 Britton J. *ABC of Smoking Cessation*. London: Blackwell, 2004.
7 Bloom BS, *et al*. Usefulness of US cost-of-illness studies in healthcare decision making. *PharmacoEconomics* 2001;19:207–13.
8 Benichou J. A review of adjusted estimators of attributable risk. *Statistical Methods in Medical Research* 2001;10:195–216.
9 Levin ML. The occurrence of lung cancer in man. *Acta Unio Internationalis Contra Cancrum* 1953;9:531–41.
10 The NHS Information Centre. *Lifestyles Statistics, Statistics on Smoking: England, 2010*. London: NHA Information Centre, 2010.

11 Twigg L, Moon, G, Walker S. *The Smoking Epidemic in England*. London: Health Development Agency, 2004.
12 Phillips CJ, Bloodworth A. *Cost of Smoking to the NHS in Wales*. Swansea: Ashwales, 2009.
13 Osborn DP, Levy G, Nazareth I, *et al*. Relative risk of cardiovascular and cancer mortality in people with severe mental illness from the United Kingdom's General Practice Rsearch Database. *Archives of General Psychiatry* 2007;64:242–9.
14 Wald NJ, Hackshaw AK. *Cigarette smoking: an epidemiological overview. British Medical Bulletin* 1996;52:3–11.
15 Hughes A, Atkinson H. Choosing Health in the South East: Smoking 2005. Oxford: South East Public Health Observatory (SEPHO).
16 Department of Health. *Health Profile of England 2007*. London: Department of Health (Health Improvement directorate, Analytical Team Monitoring Unit), 2007.
17 Hospital Episodes Statistics (HES). Hospital Episodes Statistics: Primary diagnosis. 2011. www.hesonline.org.uk.
18 The NHS Wales Informatics Service (NWIS). Health Solutions Wales, PEDW Statistics – 200910. Annual PEDW Data Tables 2011. www.infoandstats.wales.nhs.uk/page.cfm?orgid= 869&pid=41010&subjectlist=Principal+Diagnosis+%284+character+detail%29&patient coverlist=0&period=2009&keyword=&action=Search.
19 ISD Scotland. *Inpatient and Day Case Activity, Hospital Care*, 2011. www.isdscotland.org/ Health-Topics/Hospital-Care/Inpatient-and-Day-Case-Activity [Accessed 12 November 2012]
20 Health and Social Care in Northern Ireland. *Northern Ireland Hospital Statistics: Inpatient and Day Case Activity* (2010/11). www.dhsspsni.gov.uk/index/stats_research/hospital-stats/inpatients.htm [Accessed 19 November 2012]
21 Department of Health. *Payment by Results Finance and Costing Team, Reference Costs Collection Guidance 2009–10*. London: DH, 2010.
22 Department of Health. *NHS reference costs 2009–2010*. London: DH, 2011.
23 Department of Health. *National Schedule of Reference Costs Year: '2009–10' – NHS Trusts HRG Data. NHS reference costs 2009–2010*. www.dh.gov.uk/en/Publicationsandstatistics/Publications/PublicationsPolicyAndGuidance/ DH_123459 [Accessed 6 December 2012]
24 Hippisley-Cox J, Vinogradova Y. *Trends in Consultation Rates in General Practice 1995 to 2008: Analysis of the QResearch® database*. Final Report to the NHS Information Centre and Department of Health. London: The NHS Information Centre, 2009.
25 The National Audit Office. *Prescribing Costs in Primary Care*. London: The Stationery Office, 2007.
26 The NHS Information Centre. *Prescribing and Primary Care Services, Prescriptions Dispensed in the Community: England, Statistics for 2000 to 2010*. London: The Health and Social Care Information Centre, 2011.
27 Curtis L. *Unit Costs of Health and Social Care 2010*. Kent: Personal Social Services Research Unit: 2010.
28 Office For National Statistics (ONS), Statistical Bulletin: Annual Mid-year Population Estimates, 2010. Newport: ONS, 2011.
29 Welsh Government. *NHS Outpatient Activity. Health and care statistics 2011*. wales.gov.uk/topics/statistics/theme/health/nhs-outpatient/;jsessionid= T2J0T60MJGZxTJtRWptr5bNTD7YpSNKGKm2WkhNvthBF0L8LCQhn!-728126835?lang=en [Accessed 12 November 2012]
30 ISD Scotland. *Outpatient Activity, Hospital Care*, 2011. www.isdscotland.org/Health-Topics/Hospital-Care/Outpatient-Activity [6 December 2012]

31 Health and Social Care in Northern Ireland. *Northern Ireland Hospital Statistics: Outpatient activity statistics 2009/10* (revised). Belfast: Department of Health, Social Services & Public Safety, 2010.

32 Taylor D, Paton C, Kapur S. *The South London and Maudsley & Oxleas NHS Foundation Trust Prescribing Guidelines*, 10th edn. London: Informa Healthcare, 2009.

33 Health and Social Care Information Centre. *Prescription Cost Analysis England 2010*. London: Health and Social Care Information Centre, 2011.

34 *British National Formulary*. Olanzapine, 2012. www.medicinescomplete.com/mc/bnf/current/PHP18353-olanzapine-non-proprietary.htm#PHP18353-olanzapine-non-proprietary [Accessed 6 December 2012]

35 Doll R, Peto R, Wheatley K, *et al.* Mortality in relation to smoking: 40 years' observations on male British doctors. *British Medical Journal* 1994;309:901–11.

36 Doll R, Peto R, Boreham J, Sutherland I. Mortality in relation to smoking: 50 years' observations on male British doctors. *British Medical Journal* 2004;328:1519.

37 NHS HSCIC. *NHS Outcomes Framework indicators* – June 2012 Release, 2012. www.ic.nhs.uk/statistics-and-data-collections/audits-and-performance/nhs-outcomes-framework-indicators/nhs-outcomes-framework-indicators—june-2012-release [Accessed 16 November 2012]

38 McManus S, Meltzer H, Brugha T, *et al. Adult psychiatric morbidity in England, 2007. Results of a household survey*. London: The NHS Information Centre for Health and Social Care, 2009.

39 Office for National Statistics. *Population Estimates for UK, England and Wales, Scotland and Northern Ireland – mid 2009*. www.ons.gov.uk/ons/publications/re-reference-tables.html?edition=tcm%3A77–213645 [Accessed 25 January 2012]

40 American Psychiatric Association. *Diagnostic and Statistical Manual for Mental Disorders*, 4th edn (DSM-IV). Washington, DC: American Psychiatric Press, 1994.

41 Drummond M, Sculpher MJ, Torrance GW. *Methods for the Economic Evaluation of Health Care Programmes*, 3rd edn. Oxford: Oxford University Press, 2005.

42 Gray A, Clarke P, Wolstenholme J, *et al.* Applied methods of cost-effectivenesss analysis in health care. In: *Handbooks in Health Economic Evaluation*, vol 3. Oxford: Oxford University Press, 2010.

43 NICE. Guide to the methods of technology appraisal. 2008. www.nice.org.uk.

44 Cromwell J, Bartosch WJ, Fiore MC, *et al.* Cost-effectiveness of the clinical practice recommendations in the AHCPR guideline for smoking cessation. Agency for Health Care Policy and Research. *Journal of the American Medical Association* 1997;278:1759–66.

45 Parrott S, Godfrey C, Raw M, *et al.* Guidance for commissioners on the cost effectiveness of smoking cessation interventions. Health Educational Authority. *Thorax* 1998;53(suppl 5 Pt 2):S1–38.

46 West R, McNeill A, Raw M. Smoking cessation guidelines for health professionals: an update. Health Education Authority. *Thorax* 2000;55:987–99.

47 Woolacott N, Jones L, Forbes CA, *et al.* The clinical effectiveness and costeffectiveness of bupropion and nicotine replacement therapy for smoking cessation: a systematic review and economic evaluation *Health Technology Assessment* 2002;6:1–245.

48 Shearer J, Shanahan M. Cost effectiveness analysis of smoking cessation interventions. *Australian and New Zealand Journal of Public Health* 2006;30:428–34.

49 National Institute for Health and Clinical Excellence. *NICE public health intervention guidance – Brief interventions and referral for smoking cessation in primary care and other settings*. London: NICE, 2006.

50 Britton J, Edwards R.Tobacco smoking, harm reduction, and nicotine product regulation. *The Lancet* 2008;371:441–5.

51 Lawrence D, Mitrou F, Zubrick SR. Smoking and mental illness: results from population surveys in Australia and the United States. *BMC Public Health* 2009;9:285.

52 Benowitz NL, Jacob P 3rd. Daily intake of nicotine during cigarette smoking. *Clinical Pharmacology and Therapeutics* 1984;35:499–504.

53 Henningfield JE. Nicotine medications for smoking cessation. *New England Journal of Medicine* 1995;333:1196–203.

54 The Tobacco Advisory Group of the Royal College. *Harm reduction in nicotine addiction Helping people who can't quit*. London: Royal College of Physicians of London, 2007.

55 The Royal College of Physicians. *Ending tobacco smoking in Britain, Radical strategies for prevention and harm reduction in nicotine addiction*. A report by the Tobacco Advisory Group of the Royal College of Physicians. London: RCP, 2008.

56 Wang D, *et al*. 'Cut down to quit' with nicotine replacement therapies in smoking cessation: a systematic review of effectiveness and economic analysis. *Health Technology Assessment* 2008;12(2):38.

9 | Ethical and legal aspects

9.1 Context

Smoking among people with mental disorders is common; indeed, as the data in Chapter 2 demonstrate, people who report mental health symptoms are about twice as likely to smoke as people who do not. These smokers are also more likely to be heavily addicted, and to find quitting difficult. This strong association between smoking and mental disorders may reflect in part the effect of underlying common neurobiological mechanisms, but is likely to be due in much larger part to psychosocial influences. These include beliefs that smoking helps to manage the symptoms of the mental illness or the side effects of treatment for that illness, the stress and symptoms of mental illness (including the effects of stigma, relative social isolation and higher unemployment rates), more frequent exposure to others' smoke and smoking behaviours, higher rates of alcohol and other drug dependency among people with mental disorders, and the attitudes of healthcare and social work professionals towards smoking and clients.

This last, which can range from tacit acceptance and failure to challenge smoking, to endorsement or active promotion of smoking through sharing of cigarettes or other activities creating a culture of smoking, presents a particular ethical challenge. Before the Health Act 2006 was enacted, a survey found that up to a third of mental health professionals were opposed to a ban on smoking in mental health premises.[1] Mental health workers were often willing to share cigarettes with their clients and to use them as bargaining tools; cigarettes sometimes came to be used as a kind of informal currency in mental healthcare settings, much as in prisons.

Currently, where healthcare contacts happen in the home rather than in hospital, health workers may be inhibited from addressing smoking from fear of jeopardising the relationship with their patient. Where services require the patient or client to come to a clinic or other health facility, mental health workers may not wish to raise smoking from fear of putting them off attending. Where the patient is admitted or detained in a mental healthcare setting, the need to give some sense of home, privacy and independence may trump concerns with the lawfulness of smoking in a public place, the needs of others, or the physical health of the patient him- or herself. These and other considerations, which can pose conflicting ethical demands on the clinical staff involved,[2] can lead to the perpetuation of smoking in mental health settings.

9.2 Legal precedents

Several cases, finished or in progress, provide insight into the legality of extending smoke-free policies to mental health treatment settings. The case of *R(N) v Secretary of State for Health*; *R(E) v Nottinghamshire Healthcare NHS Trust* [2009] (for academic commentary see Coggon[3]) involved patients at Rampton Hospital, one of England's three high-secure forensic hospitals, who challenged the extension of the Health Act ban on smoking in public places to secure mental hospitals, which followed the expiry of the temporary exemption for these institutions under the Smoke-Free (Exemption and Vehicles) Regulations 2007 in England. (The Smoke-free Premises etc (Wales) Regulations 2007 do create an exemption for mental health premises without an expiry date. The equivalent Scottish Regulations under the Smoking, Health and Social Care (Scotland) Act 2005 also created an exemption, but a consultation was opened in 2009 on removing this.) This temporary exemption expired on 1 July 2008. The applicants argued that, as their stay in Rampton was involuntary and long term, they should be able to consider it as their home, and that extending the ban on smoking in public places to secure hospitals violated their right to a private and family life (article 8 of the European Convention on Human Rights 1950, as enshrined in the Human Rights Act 1998).

The Court of Appeal found that article 8 does not protect a right to smoke in secure mental hospitals. The reasoning of the court rested on a number of arguments, but the central premises were that, although Rampton is home like in some respects, it is nevertheless an environment with extensive restrictions on liberty, that promotion of health of both the applicants and the other residents and staff was a legitimate aim of the institution as a hospital, and that deprivation of the opportunity to smoke was neither sufficiently important as a limitation on private life nor onerous in terms of the discomfort involved as to override the legitimate aims of public health and the protection of the health of staff and inmates enshrined in the 2006 Act.

The *N* case divided the Court of Appeal, and the applicants lost on a majority decision. In the later Scottish case of *CL* (*CL v State Hospital* 2011), the judge was critical of the judgment in *N*. The *CL* case concerned regulations by the state hospital controlling the food parcels that visitors to residents of the hospitals could bring in, and a pricing policy in the hospital shop designed to encourage low-fat and low-calorie diets. *CL* partially succeeded in overturning these regulations, essentially on the ground that proper consultation had not been carried out. Although smoking is mentioned only in passing, the judgment does stress that, even in a secure hospital, the presumption needs to be that the patient has all the usual liberties with specific restrictions prescribed by law and given full justification, rather than that the patients' liberties are automatically curtailed with particular freedoms being granted ad hoc or as privileges.

At the time of writing, patients of Chadwick Lodge hospital in Buckinghamshire are petitioning the High Court to overturn a ban on smoking on hospital premises outside and off hospital premises while escorted by a nurse.[4] The news report on this case quotes a spokesman for the hospital as saying that this was a part of a healthy lifestyle policy for patients, and also that the policy followed from the *N* case. Yet whereas Rampton is a high-security hospital and smoking outside is not possible for patients there, Chadwick Lodge is a medium-security hospital and smoking outside was, until the adoption of the policy, permitted. It will be interesting to see whether the approach in the *CL* case is followed.

In the rather different context of a young offenders' institution, an inmate was unsuccessful in challenging a decision of the governor to remove his cigarettes as part of a removal of privileges as a disciplinary measure (*R(Foster) v HMP Highdown* [2010]). In the criminal justice system, unlike in the hospital system, it is clearer that many 'rights' may be granted or suspended as part of the nature of detention. However, the interesting feature of this case was that the applicant argued that the punishment was unduly severe because it imposed withdrawal symptoms upon him, and he should have been given nicotine replacement therapy (NRT). It is interesting to speculate whether, had he succeeded, the approach that mental hospitals of the medium- or low-security type could take would be to ban smoking but supply NRT as part of treatment in a more systematic way than at present. (In the case of *Shelley v United Kingdom* [2008], the issue of provision of clean needles for harm reduction in illicit opiate drug use in prison was considered, with the English courts and the European Court of Human Rights concurring that there was no obligation to provide needles. The case is discussed in Coggon.[3])

What these cases illustrate is that, from the point of view of the courts, the policies that hospitals (and prisons) may adopt to promote the health of their patients (and inmates) and protect the health of others (staff, other patients and inmates, visitors) must strike a careful balance which takes into account the overall purpose of the institution, the rights of those who live and work there, and, particularly in hospital settings, the need for careful consultation. The case law also illustrates the important fact that society at large has not reached a stable consensus on how far a smoking ban can be an important restriction on personal freedom and how far it may cause genuine distress, discomfort or suffering.

9.3 Population and individual arguments

From a population perspective, there is no good reason to think that smoking is any less important to the health of a person with a mental disorder than to anyone else, or that quitting would be any less beneficial. Given that, for more or less any health inequality that we care to consider, people with mental health problems tend to be worse off than people without, we have a rather strong reason to think that helping people with mental health problems to quit smoking would improve their general health status too. It should also help with the mental health problem itself, given what we know about the causal relationship between physical and mental wellbeing in the medium to long term. We do not have good and compelling reasons to accept the apparently common belief that smoking in people with mental health problems is unimportant relative to their mental disorder, or that smoking is or has to be part of their fragile sense of self, or that trying to help them to quit is futile or bullying.

The central ethical question is thus not at the population level; instead it is at the level of the individual client–healthcare worker and client–institution interaction. The vulnerability of patients with mental health disorders, be they in formal or informal care settings, voluntary or involuntary patients, is such that a holistic approach to their care is crucial.[5] Building and maintaining relationships is vital, as is acknowledgement of the multiple sources of stress and threats to wellbeing. Smoking will, often, be simply one source of health problems among many. It may not always be the health problem that takes priority. Yet it is not acceptable that it should *never* be a priority in the management of a given patient or group of patients. It is reasonable to expect that smoking cessation support should be included in care plans. It is not reasonable to implement an approach to smoking cessation that undermines its own objectives: a quit attempt that is the outcome of a forced choice may well fail as soon as coercion is removed (when the patient moves to a less formal environment or into the community). A homeless hostel that forbids smoking on the premises, even outdoors, may drive away some people who acutely need its help. On the other hand, it is not acceptable to sustain an environment that actively supports smoking or promotes it covertly through the support of an 'informal economy' of cigarettes, or the use of smoking rights and privileges as means by which staff may licitly or illicitly control and manage patients. It is not acceptable to manage inpatient or day-care facilities that may unwittingly encourage patients who were non-smokers or lapsed smokers to take up smoking.

A somewhat similar issue concerns the different status of informally admitted and formally admitted patients (the latter group being those 'detained under Section of the Mental Health Act'). Rules governing smoking at mental healthcare institutions will not normally differentiate between the two groups of patients. However, an informally admitted patient who finds him- or herself unable to smoke because of the institution's smoke-free policy, or because he or she cannot be accompanied outside by a member of staff, where accompaniment is thought necessary, can choose to discharge him- or herself. Seeking to do so may lead to the patient being detained formally, or to losing voluntary treatment opportunities. This presents a difficult medical ethical challenge: the need to abide by the law and the institution's policy regarding smoking, and the clinical value of helping patients stop smoking could conflict with the need to treat the presenting mental health problem as the key priority for each patient, and the need to do so without resort to coercive means, inasmuch as this is possible. A balance needs to be struck that permits a reasonably flexible approach to be taken, which encourages smoking cessation (or temporary abstinence) without resort to force or threat. Exactly how this balance is to be struck requires judgement and experience, eg taking into account the needs and welfare of staff and other patients, how far should a mental health institution seek to accommodate patients' smoking by allowing staff to accompany patients outside to smoke? And how far should institutions mitigate the effects of going outside in terms of exposure to the elements or managing security risks by building shelters or secure outdoor smoking areas? There is no precise and one-size-fits-all answer to these questions. But the central principle here is clear, which is that smoking is hazardous to health, including mental health, and a well-thought-out care plan needs to reflect best practice in smoking cessation as part of good care.

9.4 Access to treatment for smoking

Turning from policy towards clinical management of the smoking behaviour of patients, we now need to consider access to treatment by smokers with mental disorders. Starting from the obvious premise that smoking is just as important a health risk in someone with a mental disorder as it is in anyone, there is no reason to place any barriers in the way of someone who wants to quit. Thus someone with a mental disorder, in or out of formal mental healthcare, should have the same access to advice, counselling, cessation pharmacotherapies and harm reduction interventions as the general population. One troubling feature of the *Foster* case cited above is that the court did not acknowledge the difference between taking away cigarettes as removal of a privilege, and denying access to NRT as a treatment. An opportunity to help a young man to quit smoking was missed. In light of the *CL* and Chadwick Lodge cases, it appears sensible to ensure that alternative sources of nicotine are readily available, and where appropriate prescribed, for smokers obliged to abstain from smoking while in smoke-free facilities. However, as the *CL* case shows, careful consultation is needed before such policies are adopted, because nudges and incentives can be acceptable, but coercion is not.[6]

This approach does no more than suggest that we integrate smoking cessation support into mental healthcare, especially in residential settings. However, we may go further; given the evidence that we have on not only the higher prevalence of smoking in people with mental health problems but also the greater difficulties that they face in quitting, it is arguable that making treatment accessible and effective requires specific *additional* investment. The need for support is greater; the type of intervention needed may be more intensive or of longer duration. Smoke-free policies in mental health institutions, as in other public places, are justified because of the health and wellbeing of non-smoking patients and staff. The moral imperative of healthcare institutions to promote the mental and physical health of their patients (and to protect and support the mental and physical health of their staff) makes a shift in culture within mental health institutions away from one that supports smoking. But supporting smoking cessation should take note of the general approach to each patient's care. Coercion will rarely be justified. In the very specific circumstances of high-security facilities, security will necessarily take priority over patients' wishes to go outside to smoke. But applying smoke-free policies in these circumstances is not forcing patients to give up smoking for the sake of giving up smoking. Rather it is applying the necessary security measures in a situation where protecting the health and wellbeing of others (in this case through application of a smoke-free policy designed to protect others) is a priority in any case.

9.5 Summary

> - The entitlement of people with mental disorders to smoking cessation support is at least as strong as for those of the general population.
> - Their needs for such support are in many cases actually greater. Patients with mental health problems should receive at least the same level of access to smoking cessation treatment and aids to quitting as members of the general population.
> - The objectives of smoking cessation and tobacco control policies in the mental healthcare context need to take account of the complexity of the care needs of people with mental health problems.
> - The case law relating to smoking policies in formal mental healthcare settings and prisons suggests that a careful balance needs to be struck between personal rights and welfare, the objectives of the institutions, and the rights and interests of other staff and residents/inmates.
> - There is a need for greater investment in smoking cessation treatment in the mental healthcare context.
> - Smoke-free policies in mental health institutions, as in other public places, are justified on the grounds of health and wellbeing of non-smoking patients and staff.
> - The moral imperative of healthcare institutions to promote the mental and physical health of their patients (and to protect and support the mental and physical health of their staff) justifies a shift in culture within mental health institutions away from one that supports smoking.

References

1 McNally L, Oyefeso A, Annan J, *et al*. A survey of staff attitudes to smoking-related policy and intervention in psychiatric and general health care settings. *Journal of Public Health* 2006;28:192–6.

2 Lawn S, Condon J. Psychiatric nurses' ethical stance on cigarette smoking by patients: Determinants and dilemmas in their role in supporting cessation. *International Journal of Mental Health Nursing* 2006;15:111–18.

3 Coggon J. Public health, responsibility and English law: Are there such things as no smoke without ire or needless clean needles? *Medical Law Review* 2009;17:127–39.

4 *The Guardian*. Smokers win right to challenge hospital ban: Patients detained under Mental Health Act can bring test case over right to smoke outdoors. 6 May 2011. www.guardian.co.uk/society/2011/may/06/smokers-challenge-hospital-ban [Accessed 11 November 2012]

5 Silva DS. Smoking bans and persons with schizophrenia: A straightforward use of the harm principle? *Public Health Ethics* 2011;4:143–8.

6 Ashcroft RE. Personal financial incentives in health promotion: Where do they fit in an ethic of autonomy? *Health Expectations* 2011;14:191–200.

Table of cases

CL v State Hospital [2011] CSOH 21.

R(Foster) v HMP Highdown [2010] EWHC 2224 (Admin).

R(N) v Secretary of State for Health; R(E) v Nottinghamshire Healthcare NHS Trust [2009] EWCA Civ 795.

Shelley v UK Application (23800/06), [2008] 46 EHRR SE16.

10 Summary and conclusions

10.1 Smoking in Britain

Smoking is the biggest avoidable cause of death and disability in the UK. Since 1962, when the RCP published its first report on smoking and health, the prevalence of smoking in the UK has fallen dramatically: from 56% to 21% in men, and from 42% to 21% in women. This decline, which reflects the influence of increasingly effective tobacco control policies, including advertising bans, smoke-free legislation, price increases and effective, freely available smoking cessation treatment services, is now translating into substantial reductions in the annual total of deaths from smoking each year. However, the problem of smoking is far from solved. Ten million people living in the UK today are current smokers, and over 100,000 people still die every year as a consequence of their smoking. The decline in smoking has not occurred equally across all sectors of society, with the result that smoking is increasingly becoming the domain of the most disadvantaged: the poor, homeless, imprisoned and those with mental disorder. Of the many statistics in this report, two in particular stand out: first, that almost one in every three cigarettes smoked today in Britain is smoked by someone with a mental disorder; second, that over the two decades since 1993, during which the prevalence of smoking across society has fallen by a quarter, smoking rates among people with mental disorders have barely changed. The one in three cigarettes figure would be higher, if the definition of mental disorder used in this report were extended to include those dependent on alcohol or other drugs. This is a damning indictment of UK public health policy and clinical service provision.

10.2 Mental disorders and smoking in Britain

Mental disorders are common, and affect as many as one in four adults in the UK in any year, although most cases are mild and transient anxiety or depression. The more severe and enduring mental disorders, including bipolar disorder, schizophrenia and other psychoses, and severe depression are much less common, and can be severely disabling. With increasing severity of mental disorder come, among other things, progressively increased risks of social stigmatisation and marginalisation, reduced uptake or delivery of health services for physical illness, an increased risk of tobacco smoking and associated increased physical illness, and reduced life expectancy. People with mental disorders are generally around twice as likely to be smokers as those without, but smoking prevalence increases in relation to disease severity to the extent that most of those with a psychotic illness smoke. Consequently, of the 10 million smokers in the UK, up to 3 million report evidence of mental disorder, up to 2 million have been prescribed a psychoactive medication in the past year and approaching 1 million have longstanding disease. People with mental disorders are also more likely to be heavily addicted to smoking and, the more severe the mental disorder, the greater the strength of addiction. Although it is possible that mental disorder increases the risk of some physical illness independently of smoking, it is likely that the high prevalence of smoking accounts for most of the substantially lower life expectancy of people with mental disorders. In addition to reduced life expectancy, of the order of 10 years or more, smoking reduces quality of life, exacerbates poverty and adds to social stigma in this group.

10.3 The nature of the association between smoking and mental disorders

It is not clear whether the association between mental disorders and smoking is causal. Longitudinal data suggest that smokers are more likely to develop depression or anxiety disorder, and there is some evidence of common genetic determinants of both smoking and specific mental disorders, particularly depression and schizophrenia. There is also experimental evidence that nicotine can provide immediate relief from symptoms of anxiety, depression, schizophrenia and attention deficit hyperactivity disorder (ADHD), although nicotine withdrawal also creates a range of unpleasant symptoms. People with these mental disorders may therefore find that smoking helps to ameliorate symptoms in the short term, and hence be more likely to become smokers; this may explain the increased risk of smoking among people with behavioural disorders, anxiety, depression and psychosis. However, in established smokers, symptoms of nicotine withdrawal, such as depression, anxiety, irritability and agitation, mimic or exacerbate those of common mental disorders, thus perhaps accounting for at least some of the increased incidence of diagnoses of anxiety, depression and other mental disorders among people who smoke. However, further research to elucidate these associations in more detail is needed.

10.4 Smoking cessation in mental disorders

People who smoke and have mental disorders are no less likely to want to quit smoking than those without, but are more likely to be heavily addicted to smoking, more likely to anticipate difficulty quitting smoking and less likely to succeed. However, as in the general population, smokers with mental disorders are more likely to quit if provided with behavioural support and pharmacotherapy. In view of the high levels of dependence it is particularly important to provide nicotine replacement therapy (NRT) in high doses by combining slow- and faster-acting products, and provide more intensive behavioural support. Use of the non-nicotine cessation therapies, bupropion and varenicline, in people with mental disorders has been inhibited by concerns over exacerbation of depression or other adverse effects on mental health, but both therapies appear to be effective in this group and can be used, subject to supervision and monitoring to ensure that therapy is stopped in the event of adverse effects.

Quitting smoking does not markedly exacerbate mental disorders, and is likely to improve mental health symptoms over the longer term. Quitting smoking also reduces the rate of metabolism of many psychoactive drugs, doses of which therefore need promptly to be reduced, and increased in the event of relapse to smoking. Symptoms of nicotine withdrawal are easily confused with those of underlying mental disorders, and should be treated with NRT or other cessation therapy.

Smokers who are not ready or willing to attempt to quit smoking should be encouraged as strongly as possible to use NRT or other sources of nicotine to cut down on smoking, and should be provided with nicotine for smoking substitution during visits or inpatient stays in smoke-free mental health facilities.

Asking and recording smoking status, and delivery of cessation and/or harm reduction interventions to all patients who smoke, should be routine components of all primary and secondary care, including mental health services. Recent evidence suggests that ascertainment of smoking and delivery of advice to quit in primary care, where most people with mental disorders are managed, have improved in recent years in the UK, although the quality of these interventions is not known. In inpatient facilities, behavioural support and pharmacotherapy should be provided in-house.

10.5 Tobacco policy and mental health

Population-level policies to prevent smoking have contributed to significant declines in smoking prevalence across the general population over recent decades, but not among people with mental disorders. It is not clear whether this reflects a true lack of sensitivity to population policies in this group, or whether their effects are undermined (particularly in those with more severe disorder) by a pervasive culture of smoking in many mental health settings. In either case the paramount importance of all healthcare professionals taking the opportunity to address smoking in people with mental disorder is evident. Mental health facilities need to become comprehensively smoke free, in grounds as well as buildings, for all staff, visitors and patients. Abstinence from smoking, through cessation or harm reduction, needs to be established as the prevailing culture. Smoke-free policies work if comprehensive and delivered with appropriate leadership, training and support strategies for patients and staff. Investment in achieving smoke-free mental health settings, and in the support needed by patients and staff to allow this to happen, is therefore an urgent national priority.

10.6 Special circumstances

Smoking, and particularly high levels of nicotine dependence, are especially common among people admitted to forensic psychiatric facilities and for many years was culturally entrenched in the working of these facilities. Since 2007 this has changed, radically. Rampton Hospital, and subsequently all high-secure units in the UK, has successfully implemented comprehensive smoke-free policies throughout their buildings and grounds. Contrary to expectation, this has been achieved without significant adverse effects. Strong leadership, clear policies and provision of cessation support for patients and staff are among the perceived determinants of success. The experience of these institutions indicates clearly that, with similar determination, mental health facilities for the wider population with mental disorders can also become smoke free.

Smoking is also common among other population groups with a particularly high prevalence of mental disorders, including prisoners, homeless people, and people dependent on alcohol or other drugs. As in the wider mental health population, these smokers are no less likely to want to quit smoking than those in the general population, but they are more likely to be highly dependent, to be exposed to an institutional or facility culture in which smoking is engrained, and, perhaps as a result, quit attempts are less likely to succeed in this group. In drug dependence treatment facilities, addressing smoking probably improves, rather than reduces, the effectiveness of treatments for dependence on other drugs. Recent experience from New Zealand demonstrates that prisons can become smoke free, without major adverse effects, and that half of prisoners who quit smoking while in prison intend to remain non-smokers after release. Establishment of smoke-free cultures in facilities for homeless people or those with other drug dependence is likely to be equally important and effective in promoting smoking cessation. The experience of high-secure units in Britain, and prisons in New Zealand, demonstrates that such culture changes can be achieved, to widespread benefit. The National Offender Management Service for England and Wales is working towards making all prisons smoke free, although at the time of writing (February 2013) proposals to test implementation in a set of early adopter prisons, planned for spring 2013, had been postponed.

Smoking during and after pregnancy has major adverse effects on fetal and child health. Women with mental disorders are more likely to smoke throughout pregnancy, and require systematic and sustained intervention and support to maximise smoking cessation. Many children in care have mental disorders, and many smoke. It is important that child and adolescent mental health services, and local authority foster care and smoking policies, explicitly protect children from passive smoke, and provide smoke-free environments. Professionals working with or caring for young people should provide positive (ie non-smoking) role models and hence be supported to quit smoking; they should also be trained to deliver cessation advice and provide or arrange further support for children who want help to quit.

10.7 Economic costs of smoking in people with mental disorders

Smoking in people with mental disorders causes an estimated 2.6 million hospital admissions, 3.1 million GP consultations and 18.8 million prescriptions each year, at a cost of around £720m per annum. Most of this cost arises from smoking in people with anxiety or depression. Psychotropic drug costs are increased by smoking, through more rapid drug metabolism, potentially by as much as £40m per year. Preventing smoking in people with mental disorders would avoid all of these costs, and gain up to 1 million discounted and 4 million undiscounted life-years. Smoking cessation interventions and harm reduction strategies are both highly cost-effective in this population.

10.8 Ethics

People with mental disorders have an entitlement to smoking cessation support that is at least as strong as for those of the general population, but their need for support is in many cases greater. Prevention and treatment of smoking have failed this group for many years, and thus exacerbated the health inequalities sustained. It is therefore vital that patients with mental disorders receive at least the same level of access to smoking cessation treatment, and help with temporary abstinence, as members of the general population. Smoke-free policies, which help to break the culture of smoking in mental health settings, are a crucial component of this.

The objectives of smoking cessation and tobacco control policies in the mental healthcare context need to take into account the complexity of the care needs of people with mental health problems. The case law relating to smoking policies in formal mental healthcare settings and prisons suggests that a careful balance needs to be struck between personal rights and welfare, the objectives of the institutions, and the rights and interests of other staff and residents/inmates. However, policy and service provision should promote and protect health. In relation to smoking, which is the biggest preventable threat to physical health in this population, this means greater investment in smoking cessation treatment, and in establishing a smoke-free culture.

10.9 Research priorities

The findings of this report identify some clear areas of need for further research on smoking in mental health populations. Uncertainties are evident in all of the above summary statements, but some of the biggest challenges lie in understanding the mechanisms of the association between smoking and mental disorders, why people with mental disorders are more likely to be smokers and how to prevent uptake in this group, how smoking cessation support can be improved to increase cessation, how delivery of cessation interventions can be made systematic, how to maximise and maintain adherence to smoke-free policies, how to integrate harm reduction and temporary abstinence strategies into mental healthcare delivery, and how to address the needs of special groups of people with a high prevalence of smoking, such as homeless people. Where initiatives are made in these areas, it is important to include formal evaluation and reporting, as, for example, in the Rampton Hospital, for the benefit of others.

11 | Key conclusions and recommendations

Mental disorders

> - Mental disorders comprise a spectrum of conditions ranging from the mild and transient to the severe and disabling.
> - Mental disorders are common, occurring to some degree in about a quarter of adults and around 10% of children and adolescents in any year.
> - Most people with mental disorders are cared for in the community, predominantly by GPs, but also by specialist multidisciplinary teams. A minority of people with mental disorders are managed in secondary care inpatient facilities.
> - Mental disorders are associated with increased rates of a range of health risk behaviours (such as smoking, alcohol and drug misuse, poor diet, less physical activity, self-harm), poor educational and employment outcomes, homelessness, social stigmatisation, marginalisation, and reduced uptake or delivery of health services including for health risk behaviour and physical illness.
> - Life expectancy among people with many mental disorders is substantially lower than that of the general population.

Smoking among people with mental disorders

> - Smoking is around twice as common among people with mental disorders, and more so in those with more severe disease.
> - Up to 3 million smokers in the UK, 30% of all smokers, have evidence of mental disorder and up to 1 million have longstanding disease.
> - A third of all cigarettes smoked in England are smoked by people with a mental disorder.
> - In contrast to the marked decline in smoking prevalence in the general population, smoking among those with mental disorders has changed little, if at all, over the past 20 years.
> - Smokers with mental disorders are just as likely to want to quit as those without, but are more likely to be heavily addicted to smoking and to

- anticipate difficulty quitting smoking, and historically much less likely to succeed in any quit attempt.
- Over the course of a year, smokers with mental disorders are more likely to receive advice from their GP to quit smoking, and be prescribed cessation medications, but this reflects the increased frequency of their consultations. Overall, only a minority receive cessation pharmacotherapy.

Neurobiological and behavioural mechanisms linking smoking and mental disorders

- Although smoking, and high levels of dependence on smoking, are both more common in people with mental disorders, the mechanisms underlying these associations are uncertain.
- There is some evidence of common genetic determinants of both smoking and specific mental disorders, particularly depression and schizophrenia.
- Experimental evidence suggests that nicotine can relieve symptoms of anxiety, depression, schizophrenia and attention deficit hyperactivity disorder (ADHD), although nicotine withdrawal symptoms may then exacerbate symptoms of mental disorders.
- People with some mental disorders may use nicotine to ameliorate symptoms such as depression or anxiety (the self-medication model).
- However, the symptoms of mental disorders can be confused with or exacerbated by those of nicotine withdrawal, hence resulting in false attribution of relief to effects on mental disorders.
- The effects of constituents of tobacco and tobacco smoke other than nicotine on mood and cognition remain unclear.
- The association between smoking and mental disorders is therefore complex and further work is needed to help improve understanding.

Epidemiology of the association between smoking and mental disorders

- Current smoking is associated with an increased risk of onset of depression, including postnatal depression, and people with depression are more likely to become smokers.
- Current smoking is associated with an increased risk of onset of anxiety disorders, and people with anxiety disorders are more likely to take up smoking.
- Former smokers are not at an increased risk of subsequent onset of depression.
- Adolescents with eating disorders are more likely to become smokers.

- There is some evidence that people with behavioural disorders, particularly ADHD and conduct disorder, are more likely to become smokers, but no evidence that smoking increases the risk of onset of these conditions.
- There is a strong association between smoking and schizophrenia in cross-sectional studies, but longitudinal evidence on the temporal relationship is mixed.
- Adolescents with bipolar disorder may be more likely to become heavy smokers.
- Smoking is associated with an increased risk of dementia.
- People with mental disorders appear to have higher risks of cardiovascular disease and stroke (after accounting for the effects of smoking); however, there is no consistent evidence regarding an increased risk of cancer.

Smoking cessation interventions for individuals with mental disorders

- Smoking cessation interventions that combine behavioural support with cessation pharmacotherapy, and are effective in the general population, are also likely to be effective in people with mental disorders.
- Nicotine replacement therapy (NRT) is effective in people with mental disorders, but is likely to be required in high doses, for longer durations and with more intensive behavioural support than in the general population of smokers.
- Bupropion and varenicline are both effective in people with mental disorders, but should be used with appropriate supervision and monitoring; further research on their use in this population is an urgent priority.
- Smoking cessation does not exacerbate symptoms of mental disorders, and improves symptoms in the longer term.
- However, symptoms of nicotine withdrawal are easily confused with those of underlying mental disorder, and should be treated with NRT or other cessation therapy.
- Smoking cessation reduces the metabolism of some drugs, such as clozapine, used to treat mental disorder, necessitating prompt reduction in doses of affected drugs at the time of quitting, and increases in the event of relapse.
- Smokers who do not want to quit smoking, or else feel unable to make a quit attempt, should be encouraged to cut down on smoking, and to use NRT or other nicotine-containing devices (in line with the tobacco harm reduction guidance of the National Institute for Health and Clinical Excellence (NICE)) to support smoking abstinence in secondary care or other smoke-free settings, and promote the likelihood of future quit attempts.
- All primary and secondary care services should record smoking status and provide effective cessation or harm reduction interventions as a central, systematic component of care delivery. Where access to community-based

services is limited, as, for example, in secondary care settings, services should be provided in house.
> As many people with mental disorders are managed by both primary and secondary care, provision of smoking cessation support in primary and secondary care settings requires coordination to ensure consistency.
> Further research is urgently required to improve the design and content of cessation and harm reduction interventions in mental health settings, and to maximise access to and delivery of evidence-based support.

Population strategies to prevent smoking in mental disorders

> Population-level tobacco control policies have a significant effect on smoking prevalence in the general population by promoting quit attempts, and discouraging smoking uptake.
> Although specific evidence on the effect of existing population-level policies in people with mental disorders is lacking, the stability of smoking prevalence in mental health populations over recent decades in the UK suggests that they are less effective in this group.
> It may be possible to increase the impact of some approaches, such as media campaigns, by tailoring to the specific needs of mental health populations.
> However, it is also important to capitalise on the opportunities presented by contacts with mental health services to intervene to support smoking cessation and harm reduction.
> Smoking is, however, a widely accepted component of the culture of many mental health settings, making cessation more difficult for smokers.
> Smoke-free policies are a vital means of changing this culture.
> Smoke-free policies are more likely to be successful and effective if they are comprehensive, and can be implemented successfully in mental health settings with appropriate leadership and support strategies for patients and staff.
> Training and support to overcome prevailing misconceptions and negative or indifferent attitudes towards treating smoking among mental health staff are urgently needed.
> Provision of effective smoking cessation and harm reduction support for people who smoke is crucial in maintaining smoke-free policy.
> Investment in achieving smoke-free mental health settings, and in the support needed by patients and staff to allow this to happen, is therefore an urgent national priority.

Smoking and mental disorders: special circumstances

> Smoking, and particularly high levels of nicotine dependence, are especially common among people in forensic psychiatric settings and prisons, homeless people, and those with alcohol or other drug misuse.

- Smoking is also engrained in the culture of many of the institutions that care or provide for these groups.
- People in these populations are no less likely to want to quit smoking, although the likelihood of success in any quit attempt may be lower than for the general population of smokers, and smokers may also encounter obstacles to engagement with existing cessation services
- It is therefore a priority to establish smoke-free cultures and to provide suitable smoking cessation support for all smokers, particularly those with high levels of dependence, in these settings.
- Interventions to address smoking concurrently with alcohol and/or drug misuse are effective and can also support alcohol and drug abstinence.
- Women with mental disorders are more likely to smoke throughout pregnancy, but are also more likely to accept cessation support.
- Smoking cessation interventions are effective among pregnant women but may be more so if tailored to the specific needs and co-morbidities of women with mental disorders.
- Systematic and sustained intervention and support are necessary to maximise smoking cessation among pregnant women.
- Child and adolescent mental health services, and local authority foster care and smoking policies, should explicitly protect children from passive smoke, and promote smoke-free foster homes.
- Professionals working with or caring for young people should provide positive (ie non-smoking) role models and be trained to deliver cessation advice and provide or arrange further support for those who want help to quit.
- In settings where young people are most vulnerable, such as adolescent inpatient units, there should be a broad programme of health promotion aimed at preventing initiation of smoking as well as smoking cessation.
- In view of the current lack of evidence on safe, feasible and effective tobacco dependence treatment in the settings and populations covered in this book, further research is urgently required.

The economic cost of smoking in people with mental disorders

- The NHS spends approximately £720m per annum in primary and secondary care treating smoking-related disease in people with mental disorders.
- These costs arise from an annual estimated 2.6 million avoidable hospital admissions, 3.1 million GP consultations and 18.8 million prescriptions.
- Most of these service costs arise from people diagnosed with anxiety and/or depression.
- Smoking increases psychotropic drug costs in the UK by up to £40m per annum.

- Achieving cessation in 25%, 50% and 100% of people with mental disorders would, respectively, result in a gain of 5.5 million, 11 million and 22 million undiscounted life-years in the UK. At 3.5% discounting, the corresponding figures are 1.4, 2.7 and 5.4 million life-years gained.
- Harm reduction through lifelong substitution with medicinal nicotine is highly cost-effective when compared with continuing smoking, at around £8,000 per quality-adjusted life-year (QALY) gained for lifetime nicotine patch use and £3,600 per QALY for inhalators.
- Addressing the high prevalence of smoking in people with mental disorders offers the potential to realise substantial cost savings to the NHS, as well as benefits in quantity and quality of life.

Ethical and legal aspects

- The entitlement of people with mental disorders to smoking cessation support is at least as strong as that of the general population.
- Their need for such support is in many cases actually greater.
- Patients with mental health problems should receive at least the same level of access to smoking cessation treatment and aids to quitting as members of the general population.
- The objectives of smoking cessation and tobacco control policies in the mental healthcare context need to take account of the complexity of the care needs of people with mental health problems.
- The case law relating to smoking policies in formal mental healthcare settings and prisons suggests that a careful balance needs to be struck between personal rights and welfare, the objectives of the institutions, and the rights and interests of other staff and residents/inmates.
- There is a need for greater investment in smoking cessation treatment in the mental healthcare context.
- Smoke-free policies in mental health institutions, as in other public places, are justified on the grounds of health and wellbeing of non-smoking patients and staff.
- The moral imperative of healthcare institutions to promote the mental and physical health of their patients (and to protect and support the mental and physical health of their staff) justifies a shift in culture within mental health institutions away from one that supports smoking.

Overall conclusions

- Smoking is extremely common in people with mental disorders, causing major reductions in life expectancy and quality of life, exacerbating poverty and presenting major economic costs to the NHS and wider society.

- Despite consuming a large proportion of tobacco in the UK and being heavier smokers, only a minority of people with mental disorders receive effective smoking cessation interventions.
- Prevention and treatment strategies to date have made little if any impact on smoking in this population.
- This failure does not arise from substantially lower motivation among smokers with mental disorders to quit smoking.
- It is likely that the persistent acceptance of smoking as a normal behaviour in primary and secondary care, and failure by health professionals to address smoking prevention as a health priority, drives and perpetuates the high prevalence of smoking in people with mental disorders.
- This persistent high prevalence of smoking reflects a major failure of public health and clinical services to address the needs of a highly disadvantaged sector of society.
- There is a moral duty to address this problem in the future, and to prioritise the rights of people with mental disorders to the same protection and health interventions as the general population
- Smoke-free policy is crucial to promoting smoking cessation in mental health settings.
- All healthcare settings used by people with mental disorders should therefore be completely smoke free.
- Smokers with mental disorders using primary and secondary care services, at all levels, should be identified and provided routinely and immediately with specialist smoking cessation behavioural support, and pharmacotherapy to relieve nicotine withdrawal, promote cessation and reduce harm.
- Commissioners should require mental health service settings to be smoke free, and to provide support for cessation, temporary abstinence and harm reduction.
- Service indicators, such as the primary care Quality Outcome Framework (QOF) and Commissioning for Quality and Innovation (CQUIN), should measure and incentivise cessation, not just delivery of advice to quit.
- All professionals working with or caring for people with mental disorders should be trained in awareness of smoking as an issue, to deliver brief cessation advice, to provide or arrange further support for those who want help to quit and to provide positive (ie non-smoking) role models. Such training should be mandatory.
- There is no justification for healthcare staff to facilitate smoking.
- Research funding agencies should consider encouraging and investing in research to address this major cause of ill-health, and health inequalities, in British society.